Advance Reviews

"Chris writes with grace. And from what I can tell, he has lived with grace despite the pain, heartache and indignities of his cruel disease. His story of a life awfully altered, and yet so purposefully lived is deeply touching. Every page is a moving reminder of the meaning of the human spirit."

> — Bob Costas, long-time sportscaster, media host and author

"Honest, moving story of how one family and their community changed the world of ALS and healthcare advocacy. Chris and Christine share deep life lessons that can help all of us, no matter the circumstances. A must read!"

> — Merit Cudkowicz, MD, Chief of Neurology Massachusetts General Hospital; Julieanne Dorn Professor of Neurology Harvard Medical School

"This is a wonderful memoir written by a man with the greatest spirit and commitment. In the face of such unexpected and devastating adversity, a diagnosis of ALS, Chris Pendergast shows us how a committed and kind human being can change the world- from friends, to patients then on to researchers that he touched and who had the opportunity to get to know. His writings allow us all to glimpse into the man behind this valuable, compassionate mission. Good luck with the book!"

— Jeffrey D. Rothstein MD, PhD, The John W. Griffin Director of the Brain Science Institute; Professor of Neurology and Neuroscience; Director, Robert Packard Center for ALS Research, Johns Hopkins University, School of Medicine

"Chris Pendergast is an American treasure. His courage and grace in the face of adversity is truly heroic. His passion for education has always been his trademark as he has made an indelible mark on the fight to find a cure for ALS. For more than two decades, he's inspired me and thousands of others. I recommend that you read about his journey because he will inspire you, too."

— David Cone, former Major League Baseball pitcher, current commentator for the New York Yankees

Blink Spoken Here

Blink Spoken Here

Tales from a Journey to Within

Dr. Christopher Pendergast
& Christine Pendergast

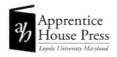

Apprentice
House Press
Loyola University Maryland

First Edition

Hardcover ISBN: 978-1-62720-256-5
Paperback ISBN: 978-1-62720-257-2
Ebook ISBN: 978-1-62720-258-9

Printed in the United States of America

Acquisitions & editing by Isabella De Palma
Cover design by Chelsea McGuckin
Promotion plan by Isabella De Palma

Published by Apprentice House Press

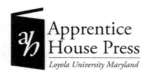

Apprentice
House Press
Loyola University Maryland

Apprentice House Press
Loyola University Maryland
4501 N. Charles Street
Baltimore, MD 21210
410.617.5265
www.ApprenticeHouse.com
info@ApprenticeHouse.com

Dedication

We dedicate this book to each other. Elvis Presley prophetically crooned our wedding song in his smash release, *The Wonder of You*. Indeed, we gave each other consolation, hope and strength to carry on.

We were fortunate to have met and loved one another. We both agree, we blessed the day we found "us" as the Everly Brothers sang in the hit, *Let It Be Me*.

Our marriage brought two kind, compassionate and productive children, Melissa and Christopher, who have been there for us from the beginning. Our grandson Patrick brought renewed gratitude and joy.

This story is a testament to our commitment, resilience and love in the face of adversity.

Foreword

by Jonathan Eig

I once tried to imagine what Lou Gehrig would have said if he had been healthy enough in 1939 to travel to Cooperstown, New York, for his induction in baseball's Hall of Fame. I visualized him saying these words that I wrote:

It is a wonderful honor to gain induction today to the Baseball Hall of Fame and to join the pantheon of great athletes and great men who have come before me. This game of baseball has meant everything to me, as it has so many boys. It took me and my family out of poverty. It taught me to be a man. I'm proud that I played hard and that the Yankees won a lot of ballgames and our share of World Series with me at the first sack. I'm proud I hit the ball square and sometimes far. I'm proud that I played fair. I'm proud that I showed my opponents the same respect I showed my own teammates. I'm proud I gave it my all every time I grabbed a bat or slipped on a glove.

But I guess if there's one thing above all else that I'm proud of, one thing that made me who I am today and got me to the Hall of Fame, it would be this: strength.

Yes, strength. You see, I was a poor kid, a little on the pudgy side. I didn't have much confidence in myself. My mother loved me so much she didn't want to ever let me leave the house. I had three siblings who died, and I was her last hope. So I grew up shy and nervous. I never thought I would amount to much. But my father, he taught me the value of exercise, and soon I started packing on muscle. I was the biggest and strongest kid on the block, and then I was the biggest and strongest kid in high school, and after that in college. And I began to believe in myself. To walk into a clubhouse and see Babe Ruth and Bob Meusel and Waite Hoyt wearing Yankee uniforms and welcoming you to the club, boy, you'd better believe in yourself. That's the first thing I tell kids today when they ask me how to be a ballplayer. I tell them it's not about how you swing the bat or grip the ball. First thing you have to do is believe. Second thing you have to do is work hard. If you do those things, even if you don't amount to much of a ballplayer, you're going to be OK.

Me, I turned out to be a pretty fair ballplayer. I have a lot of people to thank for that, including my parents, my beautiful wife, my coaches, my teammates, the owners of the Yankees, and, of course, the fans. You probably heard that I gave a speech at Yankee Stadium when I found out I was sick…that I was… dying…I said I considered myself the luckiest man on the face of the earth. Well, I wasn't saying I was lucky to get this disease, this amyotrophic lateral sclerosis. Nobody's lucky to get sick. I was saying I was lucky to have had a good life, lucky to have parents and a wife who love me, lucky to have played baseball. Mostly, I guess I was lucky to be strong. But here's what I've learned, now that this disease has got me behind in the count no balls and two strikes: I learned that it's not really muscles that make you strong.

I learned that it's how you face a challenge—like how my parents faced the challenge of losing three kids, or how my wife is facing the challenge of losing me...

I hit some balls pretty hard in my day, and I suppose that did take a kind of strength. But hitting a baseball doesn't make a man a hero. There are a whole lot of people out there as sick as I am, people with ALS and all kinds of other diseases. They're not giving up. They're meeting every day head on, still swinging for the fences with everything they've got.

To fight on through disaster, to dedicate your final days to the loved ones you will soon leave behind, and to believe in yourself when you have nothing left but that will to believe...that is the greatest strength I know.

Thank you.

As Lou Gehrig's biographer, I feel a responsibility to speak up for Lou and to share his story, and even to put words in his mouth from time to time. But the beautiful irony is that I really don't have to because Chris Pendergast has carried on Gehrig's legacy so bravely and so well.

Chris and I met in 2006 at Johns Hopkins University in Baltimore, where I had been invited to address scientists working on a cure for ALS. I said that day that I believed ALS would be cured in my lifetime. I still believe that. But I also pointed out, sadly, that Lou Gehrig had believed it, too, when he was diagnosed in 1939.

Gehrig's story is the stuff of tragedy—baseball's strongest man inflicted with a fatal disease that wore his muscles away. But there's beauty in it, too, because the disease is forever linked to a man whose courage and optimism grew as his physical strength faded. Gehrig chose not to hide his illness from the public. He chose not to seek pity. He called himself "the luckiest man on the face of the earth" and meant it. And his courage proved contagious. He has inspired millions of people facing hardship to hold their heads high and to concentrate on what life has given them rather than what might be taken away.

In *Blink Spoken Here: Tales from a Journey to Within,* Chris shows he is a worthy heir to the Gehrig line. He may have Lou Gehrig's disease, but he also has Lou Gehrig's strength, Lou Gehrig's love, and Lou Gehrig's hope. To read his story is to share that strength, that love and that hope.

Jonathan Eig is the author of *Luckiest Man: The Life and Death of Lou Gehrig.*

Introduction

It was not a dramatic event like a building collapse but more a steady deterioration similar to bridge failure. I was imploding. In 1993, my physical presence began shrinking before my very eyes. My contact with the world was severing, one function at a time. Angry, scared and saddened I was like a stubborn mule fighting with tenacity for each inch I surrendered. First it was dressing, followed by grooming, driving, toileting, walking, feeding, and breathing. Now I cling to my last vestiges of talking. It forced me to retreat towards within. The exterior husband, father, and friend was left behind.

Rene Descartes said, "*I think, therefore, I* AM!"

Even though now deep within, let there be no doubt. "Though I am statuesque in appearance, I am still flesh and blood. I am not a vegetable to be stored or pitied. Don't ignore me by talking to my wife as if I cannot understand." I proclaimed.

"My husband is a man with ALS, he is normal in every other way," Christine tells people.

Amyotrophic lateral sclerosis (ALS) is a devastating neuromuscular disease. By misfortune, it selected me as one of its victims. My life changed forever with the diagnosis. I felt compelled to write about my experiences and thoughts living with this unwelcomed interloper. When I shared some of my work, people's reactions were universal: write a book. I dismissed the notion as obligatory flattery. I continued trying to live and work teaching with my grim companion rather than resign to accept the death it promised. As I did, I wrote. First, I typed normally on my knock-off Apple II e, then with an adaptive device allowing my hands and arms to glide over the keyboard. Following many years, I graduated to use a head mouse controlled by infrared reflective dots taped on my forehead to choose the letters. Finally, I resorted to the eye-controlled device I use today.

Time passed, our path zigzagged, the number of stories grew and the accolades amplified. My writings eventually morphed into this book. My wife helped me write it with honesty and frankness about this brutal killer. I told the joys and blessings it brought us. I talked of hope and faith. I also revealed the terror, worry and torment it wrought on our family. These writings comprised our life experience for the past twenty-five years. To the best of our memory, they are accurate with my wife providing much of the specific details.

I divided its forty-four chapters into two sections, one reflections and stories from my personal life in the order I was inspired to write them. The second part chronologically details our advocacy work beginning with a fifteen-day wheelchair odyssey from Yankee Stadium to Washington, D. C. This section explains raising over eight million dollars and founding the ALS Ride for Life organization.

Aside from receiving the diagnosis of Lou Gehrig's disease, *The ALS Ride for Life* is another of my life's seminal events. Stretching over the last quarter century, it began with the Ride to Congress in 1998, launching my public advocacy life. I have been riding my chair ever since, over 3,000 miles.

I was born to be a teacher. I hope our book informs and inspires the reader. My wife and I will continue trying to cope and live productive, happy lives with our children and grandson. In the process, I will continue to teach.

Part One

Stories and Reflections From Our
Personal Lives

Celebrating Life

I wrote and named this poem for my Principal shortly after I returned to work after my diagnosis in 1993. I tried to capture my thoughts about God's role in life, patience and ultimate acceptance. I hope he recalled it years later, when it was his turn to die. I hope that it brought him peace.

L'Chaim

Look! See the gossamer threads of our life sway to and fro.
They dance with the winds of fate. Sinuous wisps of ourselves:
writhing in unrehearsed undulation. Mystical and incompre-
hensible, they swirl about.

Introspectively, we strain to see their meaning.
We view them in a moment, a frozen frame. But, this very act
errantly halts the procession. Peering into time, stuccoed and
fixed, the strands lose their fluid rhythm.

Thus exposed, we can see only a tangled web of life's travail.
Painful and disparate.
Fear not.......but take heart.

*This Gordian knot is but a moment's twist of our gossamer
threads.*

*The MASTER is working the loom, weaving the threads.
With patterns unfolding, it will become the beautiful mosaic of
our LIFE.*

*Err not then! Look not and see only bare strands.
Look beyond, transcend the moment.
See the dance of the gossamer threads: beauty, harmony, and
peace
In His time the weave will reveal its design; Clarity prevails and
serenity abides.*

Besides Christine (and of course, my mental health therapist, Dr. Philip Melnekoff), Gary was my closest confident. I met him when he became my supervisor as the Director of Special Services in our school district in the late 80's. We were nothing alike physically. He was slender and slightly built. Gary was an impeccable dresser, usually sporting a jacket and tie. Most often, I was in jeans and maybe a flannel shirt. The only characteristic we shared were our beards. Even then, his black one was neatly cropped short while my reddish-brown one was long and wild - more like a mountain man than an administrator.

We were the same age and shared similar educational values. I liked him a lot. We clicked and worked well together. Dr. Burns, his official title, received an appointment as Principal of my school several years afterward. Working every day together, we grew closer.

4

His support during my long process of diagnosis was encouraging and helpful. When the crushing news of my diagnosis came, he became a rock for me.

"Take as much time as you need, Chris, everything will be taken care of for you," he told me over the phone.

I sobbed back, "Thank you, Gary."

In two days after finding out, I wanted to return to work. It was a diversion from reality. I loved my work and it was a joy to be with my kids. My return was emotional. Everyone knew my fate. It must have been a heartbreaking scene for everyone. A beloved teacher comes back for his final hurrah. He was going down fighting.

I bravely entered back into reality going back days after receiving my diagnosis of ALS, aka Lou Gehrig's disease. I went directly to the office.

Gary and I hugged tight and long. I cried in his arms, "I didn't want this,"

"Nor did I. What will you do?" he asked.

"I'll teach," I responded.

"Are you sure that's what you want to do," he continued to question.

A flash went through me. Not normally an outspoken or presumptuous man, I said something quite out of character.

"Before I got sick, I taught about living." I said to him. "Now, I will teach about how to die."

He looked at me shaking his head in agreement. Gary knew me well. He understood my point.

"There are no lesson plans written for this unit, so don't be looking for one during my yearly observation and evaluation," I said with a sardonic smile. "I'll have to improvise and figure it out as I go."

With Gary's help, I taught through my growing disabilities. He facilitated every modification I required to enable me to continue teaching. He was an ardent supporter of my first Ride to Washington in '98. I could not ask for anything more from a boss.

Tragically, Gary developed cancer over that summer. Gary did not return in the fall; he was too sick. He did not respond to treatment. The disease traveled at warp speed. In a cruel turn of events, we both became *Dead Men Walking*.

His disease progressed fast. I now became his encourager. I visited him in the hospital hours before he died. I think of him often and with grateful fondness.

The lesson I learned from this was life must not be viewed in isolation or in a narrow slice. By doing so a distorted image is created. If a circle were examined closely, it appears to be a series of random straight lines. To get the true image, one must step back and view it in its entirety. Only then does the true design reveal itself. The same is true with life.

How Soon Is Soon?

In my eyes, teaching was not something I did to earn a living. It was more an extension of who I was and how I lived. My mind thirsted to know and understand the marvels of our glorious world. Learning was living. Living was learning. What better endeavor than to co-discover and share the mysteries of the universe? I was a student of life. Teaching these marvels came second nature to me.

By age forty-four, my educational career was in high gear, honed by years of experience. I ran an award-winning science center filled with all sorts of incredible things including numerous scaled, finned, feathered and furred creatures. I created an intellectual version of Toys R Us, a room to captivate young minds. By all external measures, I was a successful and esteemed elementary teacher. I loved my job and it loved me.

Reverberation rumbled through the school and beyond into the community after the news leaked out about my diagnosis. When I returned responses were hushed because I did not go public with my devastating news. It is understandable, I was unapproachable for a while searching for my way to cope with my fatal future. Showing me respect, everyone waited for a signal before broaching the subject with me.

As I grew in understanding and acceptance, I returned to the joys of life. I eased back into myself. I returned to living. I smiled and sang once more as I walked on campus. My classroom breathed again. I remained silent in public.

Seven months later, during ALS Awareness Month in May, I found enough strength to write an opinion piece for a major suburban newspaper, *Newsday*. For the first time, I revealed my fatal disease, ALS. I described the deplorable state of research and called for more attention to the illness. Coming out was cathartic as I told the readers I will die. I breathed easier without the weight of secrecy on my shoulders. The article demonstrated my refusal to 'go quietly into the night and chose instead to rage against the light'. To use a baseball metaphor, I intended to go down swinging. The piece appeared on a Friday afternoon. I held my breath and braced for the unknown reactions.

The trepidation after writing the piece did not last long. On the Monday following the article's publication, I stood in front of my school awaiting the bus as normal. The youngsters filed off and looked everywhere but at me. There was no joy in Mudville.

My position was teaching the gifted program for elementary students from a large district in Northport, Long Island. My oversized classroom at Dickinson Ave. School served as a magnet school. Busses brought children from their home schools to work with me in the Habitat Science Center. Since the children were young, I met and escorted them across campus to the room. The five-minute walk was a relaxed and spontaneous time for chatter, news and extemporaneous lessons suiting the moment. As we walked to the classroom that day the line began to stretch out and I found myself straggling near the end.

One of my third graders walking with me, Jimmy DeVerna called "Mr. P!" I turned and bent towards him to give him my full attention as we walked. My posture invited him to continue. "My mother told me you are sick," he declared.

"I am, Jimmy." To reassure him, and perhaps myself, I quickly added, "but I am doing well."

"She said you're gonna die." It was clear the family discussed my illness. Jimmy heard his mother talking about my prognosis and the fact that survival time is short. "Will it be soon?" he inquired in a rising voice.

This crucial question spoke to me as a patient and not a teacher. I did not want to lie nor could I tell him the brutal adult truth that I would be dead in a couple of years because ALS is untreatable and unstoppable. I didn't want to evade him but I didn't want to overwhelm him either. With steps left before the two of us entered the classroom, I slowed our pace to a crawl, buying time to come up with an answer.

As an undergraduate, I studied the foundations of education. Socrates, one of the greatest of all teachers, perfected the art of teaching through questioning. I learned if you ask the right question, you will find the right answer. The teacher inside me finally spoke, framing my answer for him as a question. "Well, Jimmy, what do you mean by soon?" I gave him time and waited for him to think.

With innocence and honesty, he raised his eyebrows, widened his eyes, hunched his shoulders and spoke. "I donno, maybe a couple of weeks?" he replied. I laughed to myself, half with surprise and half with relief. He provided me with the answer.

His reply helped me compose an answer dictated to him and his point of reference. I rested my hand on his shoulder, smiled and looked straight at his face. "Oh Jimmy, you don't have to worry about me dying soon. I promise you, I am going to be here a long, long time!" I declared with a teacher's authority. He accepted my answer. His angst eliminated, he stepped into the classroom, back into the innocent world of eight year olds. I followed him into the room, a teacher once more. The patient remained at the door.

Over the next two years, I looked at Jimmy and relived that moment many times. He graduated elementary school and we said our goodbyes. Six years later, Jimmy graduated high school. The following year, I retired, closing a three-decade career. I lost contact with him but know he graduated college. Over the ensuing years, I have used Jimmy's story quite often to convey my wonder about the vaporous essence of time. Time is an enigma.

My diagnosis forced me to consider the grim reality. I did not want to die "soon" and I didn't mean a couple of weeks. I imploringly prayed to escape the statistics. I hoped to live beyond ALS's cruel expectations: death within thirty-six months.

This past Columbus Day weekend brought an extraordinary anniversary. With it, I began my twenty-seventh year of learning, marveling and teaching about the mysteries of the universe. I kept my promise to Jimmy. A mystery to me is how I have kept it for so long.

I continue to pray. I still hope for tomorrows. I look forward to many more awe generating explorations. There are more mysteries still to ponder. Who knows, perhaps I may even still teach.

The lesson I learned from this was how time is, indeed relative. ALS, like any terminal illness alters how time is measured. A lifetime becomes compressed into the course of the disease. You are not guaranteed anything, even the prognosis. Life each day to the fullest and hope for tomorrows.

Deadly Déjà vu

The pain was significant and seemed so innocent at first.

I reassured myself, "Who doesn't get an occasional cramp?" The beginning symptoms did not raise any red flags. Oblivious to the warning signs, I spent many nights walking the hall trying to work out a Charlie-horse that struck during a peaceful sleep. The bad ones forced me to double over in pain as my insolent leg refused to support my weight. In time, these unwanted contractions spread into muscles I did not know I had.

My struggles not to ram the car in front of me often interrupted the endless bumper-to-bumper work commute. Writhing in pain, I arched up, rising clear off my seat to stretch my torso so an abdominal cramp would ease. Other times I resembled an opera star exercising my neck, mouth and facial muscles before a performance. My chin rose so high I had difficulty seeing the road when I stretched throat muscles conspiring to choke me. These must have been peculiar sights to the drivers traveling alongside my car. I can imagine what they were thinking as our eyes locked during the snail-paced drive. If it happened now in the era of ubiquitous cell phones, someone would call the police and report a DWI.

My odd mixture of symptoms pushed me to my family doctor.

"What brings you today," he questioned.

"I have been getting these weird kind of cramps, Doctor."

He probed deeper, "In one muscle or an area?"

"Well, I get them everywhere." I told him. I went on with the specifics.

He wanted to know, "Has anything changed in your diet? Do you do anything new, like working out?"

"Nothing out of the ordinary," I detailed my weekend warrior lifestyle of chopping wood, mixing cement, digging holes, shingling roofs and a myriad of other jobs over-ambitious homeowners tackle. He listened, put a stethoscope to my lungs, palpated my abdomen and drew blood. He tested my heart.

"Things look okay," he announced. "Let's get your lab work back and we'll go from there. See me in two weeks."

It turned out my EKG was good as was the other lab work. I had a slight elevation of sugar level. However, the weight scale told another tale. I had become middle-aged plump. The doctor reminded me I turned forty, was out of shape and held a sedentary job.

"How do you expect your body to respond to the abuse you inflict on it," he asked. "You have to take better care of yourself." He sent me home with orders to clean up my lifestyle: lose weight, exercise with more regularity, eat a healthier diet and get proper rest. To ease my transition to this healthier and with hope, cramp-free lifestyle he suggested, "Drink tonic water. It has quinine in it. Quinine will help the cramping."

Like most, I had partial success with my lifestyle changes. Regardless of my efforts, the cramping continued. Seeking relief from the agonizing muscle spasms, I graduated from tonic water to over the counter quinine pills. There were no improvements and my gyrations became fodder for fun at family gatherings. Little did anyone suspect the disaster occurring just inches under my skin. The twitching was symptomatic of an impending nerve Armageddon. Unbeknownst to me, my nerves were fighting a losing battle, overwhelmed by a mysterious force. The twitches were their last ditch efforts to survive.

Several years later the tipping point came, pun intended. I began falling. Once it was over my son's bicycle that I tried to step over. Another was during a lumberjack impersonation as I chain-sawed some trees on my property. As I tumbled off the log I was standing on, the buzzing blade brushed the leg of my jeans, shredding it. It nearly took my leg off. My symptoms were getting worse.

When I pointed out to my wife how my muscles twitched once, we stared in amazement. My skin dimpled and danced.

"It looks like leprechauns jumping on it, "she exclaimed.

It was a bizarre sight. Although not painful, it was difficult to watch the waves of chaotic movement ripple across my body parts. It was apparent, things were not normal, but I thought still benign.

Upon a return visit to my GP, he recommended a neurologist. When I went for that visit, he took a medical history. "I understand from your family doctor you are having fasciculations?" I nodded in agreement. "Let's take a look at you." With that, he raised his stethoscope.

He performed a physical exam. The twitching began, almost on demand. "Do you mind if I call my partner in to see this?" he said in a surprised tone.

He stepped out of the room. Rather than be alarmed, I was relieved my symptoms were of sufficient interest to warrant another view. They looked, pointed, nodded and hmmmmed.

Growing concerned at their reactions, I interrupted the viewing by asking, "Doctor, what was causing them?"

His voice replied with assurance, "There are many possibilities, in all likelihood something benign. Most of them are." He scheduled a follow up visit to do an electromyogram or EMG.

I arrived at the office not knowing much about the test I was about to take. I was unfamiliar with the procedures. I assumed it was like an EKG. God was I wrong. He explained the test measures electrical impulses within the nerve.

"With it, I see the health of the nerve. First we'll take some measurements."

He stretched a tape measure down my forearm and made marks as guides. He looked like a tailor measuring my arm for a suit. At the end of his marks, he taped electrodes to register an electrical impulse. Next, he brought out the machine. It looked like a Hollywood prop from a Frankenstein movie: A gadget to reenergize the dead.

I opened my eyes wider when he took out needles that reminded me of what an acupuncturist may use. They were several inches long. He connected them to the machine with thin wires.

He stated. "I need to insert these into your muscle fibers." Then, his Franken-machine would generate voltage to course down the nerve.

"Oh, I see," was all I could muster as I sat with no protest, submitting to the procedure. The tingling, pulsing surge of electricity shot down my arm multiple times. It felt unusual, uncomfortable but not quite painful. It was more surprising than anything else was. I wondered how it would feel to be electrocuted, every muscle at one time? He did a few different muscles.

The test did not rattle me until he looked me in the eyes and instructed, "Stick out your tongue."

With nonchalance, he grasped the tip of my tongue, pulled it out until it hurt. Holding it snug in tweezers, he skewered the center and back with several probes. Once he had them all in, he gave me the ridiculous order.

"Now relax," he told me.

I smile now imagining all of the stuff dangling from my quivering tongue. Relax? I did my best to comply with his instructions to relax and keep my tongue still.

The test ended, thank goodness. He drew blood and prescribed an array of exotic tests done searching for immune disorders or another explanation. After the visit, I found myself wandering in the public library reference room thumbing through medical books to find out what he was looking for with the tests. The ailments I uncovered went from stark to grim. As I identified one after another. I realized I could be a very sick man.

Several weeks went by as I waited. I called a couple of times to monitor the status of the tests. I grew more concerned with each passing day. Columbus Day fell on October 13 and schools were off making a long weekend. Every other teacher was delighted. There was no joy in my home as I grew anxious awaiting some news. By afternoon, the cloudy autumn day turned cold and rainy.

The anticipated call came that day in the early evening. I bantered with the doctor as I summoned up my courage. I started, "So doctor, have any of my tests come back?"

"Yes, all of the tests came back negative." For the moment, I was relieved. I pressed him for an explanation for my symptoms.

After a few evasive exchanges for my questions, he concluded, "You should come back in a couple of months and we can check you again,"

"Why is that?" I wanted to know what he was looking for and what would change in a couple of months. I continued seeking something specific.

"Well, your EMG shows some nerve degeneration," he replied in a general, open way saying nothing.

"Nerve degeneration? Really? That doesn't sound so good." He mumbled something about different possibilities. He said he was not sure of the cause. I pushed him to answer the question, "What do you think is going on?"

His answer was a question. "Mr. Pendergast, have you ever heard of Lou Gehrig's Disease?"

I did. I knew where he was going. After that, I don't remember anything. I was numb from Lou Gehrig's disease reverberating in my head like the sound of gunshot fired next to my ear. It ricocheted through my head. I hung up and broke down.

Struggling to breathe, I told my wife. Christine and I held each other close and our nestled faces moistened from each other's tears. Life as we knew it was over. I was 44 years old.

The rain struck the kitchen windows streaking downward to match the tears streaming down our faces.

Because of the research I had done, it wasn't as if I was surprised. I shared with my wife before the call that my symptoms appeared to be ALS. The confirmation was still devastating.

My family was precious, my career noble: I had a good life, everything considered. I realized I was content. I wanted to continue for as long as possible doing almost the same thing. I stayed home a couple of days to let it all sink in. Thursday I returned to work, anxious to re-enter the world of normalcy.

Teaching was my therapy and I threw myself into it. My colleagues were told about my diagnosis before I came back. They surrounded me in a loving, protective cocoon. I was glad to be there doing what I loved.

One icy January afternoon in 1994, I escorted my students to the bus as usual. After they boarded, I returned to my classroom. On the walkway back, I failed to negotiate an ice patch and slipped. I fell hard, hitting my head, knocking me unconscious for a moment. I laid motionless sprawled out on the sidewalk. The children in the neighboring classrooms saw me. Their teacher called the office. I felt groggy when I attempted to stand, but could not. I looked up to see the angelic face of our school nurse, Maureen, dispatched to rescue me.

"Chris, stay there a minute until you feel strong. You took a bad fall. There is no blood, so nothing was cut." She spoke as if I was a routine visitor to her school office. Maureen Conroy was a gentle soul with a warming smile and soft voice.

Her personality suited her role as surrogate mother to the 500 children in her care.

Her calm manner helped me as well. Not much over five feet, many fifth graders towered above her. With some assistance from her, I arose. She struggled to steady me. I was in a daze and wobbled from side to side.

"You are cold Chris. I want to get you back inside your classroom. Don't rush, Chris, take your time. Here, lean on my arm."

We looked like the odd couple as my six-foot-plus frame leaned on her petite, five-foot body.

"Easy does it, Chris," she warned as we went back. I walked on automatic pilot.

As the fog lifted, I realized I did not know who or where I was. The woman standing next to me holding my arm was a stranger. In a soothing manner, she said conversational things like the weather and the ice.

"It has been cold. There is ice everywhere. Kids are coming in all day long from falls."

Maureen calmed me by talking. Once safe inside my room, she eased me into my chair and sat across from me. She answered the questions I peppered at her. My principal came to check on me. She assured both of us the bump was just temporary.

"He is ok. His memory will return in short order," she said.

She was right. The presence of my principal alone helped jog my vague memories. He left after being satisfied I was okay. Maureen spent the better part of an hour coaxing me back to reality.

I began to remember details about my life, but something eluded recollection. I had a haunting and ill-defined premonition. I knew not all was well but I didn't understand why. Somehow, I sensed Maureen was not disclosing everything. I held a menacing feeling that I could not shake.

I grew agitated for the first time since losing my memory. My paranoia was palpable as I raised my voice.

I quizzed her, "What are you holding back? Why won't you tell me?" I grew mean and bordered on abusive. I was so agitated. "Maureen, something is missing. Please tell me!" I pleaded with her.

"Everything is okay, Chris, don't be upset. Try to calm yourself." Her eyes contradicted her words. There was something more.

I shouted, "You are not telling me the truth." I stood up and demanded to know what she was holding back. My memory was shielding me from something terrible. I could see it in her face.

Maureen saw my dismay and she was not able to calm me down. She took my hand in hers and told me to sit down. Looking into my soul, she stroked my hand and began to speak.

"Chris, you don't remember you are sick, do you?"

The words terrified me. Angry, I pulled away and stood up. I looked at her, "Just tell me what the hell is going on."

Unable to avoid it any more, she blurted, "Chris, I am sorry, you have ALS."

Stunned, every other question troubling me evaporated. "A L S?" I forced out the letters. She looked directly at me and nodded in affirmation. Her revelation was shocking and new. There was no memory of my diagnosis.

For the second time I heard, "You have ALS."

I lowered my six-foot-two frame into the small student desk next to her as I tried to digest her words. They opened a floodgate of emotion once more. I reeled from the news. This time I understood the implication. In an instant, I went from a confused, agitated man to a heartbroken one. I hunched over in my seat, put my face in my hands closed my eyes and cried. She extended her arm and clasped my hand again.

In the darkness, I heard sobbing. Maureen cried with me. Her muffled sobs soothed my aching heart. I knew I was not alone.

Life is not fair or unfair. Life just is. Most people in middle age never have to hear the devastating news, "You have a terminal illness." Others like me are not so lucky. It is a breath stealing, mind-altering experience. Readers who have experienced it comprehend what I mean. Those untouched by a harbinger of death cannot fathom it. They can only empathize.

I went through that rite of passage once. How could it ever happen again? A diagnosis of ALS is a statistical rarity. Yet, it did. Worse, the second time I received the news was as terrible as the first. The double diagnosis scenario has to be one for the record book.

Life is too short to spend wishing things were not so. Things are what they are. Some occurrences are not our choice. However, we do choose how to respond. We decide how to live the life we get.

I said my second diagnosis was simply, "A deadly déjà vu."

The lesson I learned from this was the importance of empathy. One supportive person is all it takes to transition safely through a crisis. Each of us will be presented with an opportunity to support someone in crisis. I learned just how much value there is in taking that opportunity.

Oh, The Games We Played

I always remembered the game with fondness. No birthday party seemed complete unless they played it. In my childhood mind, it held a riveting power. When I played so long ago, I used to alternate between titillating excitement and ominous dread. Where would I find myself when the music stopped?

The days came as a young parent, when I hosted my own group of excited youngsters at the birthdays of my children. Of course, they played musical chairs. The game was not the same for me. No longer caught in the intrigue as a player, I could stand back and observe. A generation ago, the faces were playmates. Now I saw just players. How different that game had become.

The stereo spun birthday records. The music blared through our small living room as they began their game.

"Are you ready?" my wife slowly asked the impatient kids. Then she put the record player on to begin the music.

I studied them as they played with childhood innocence. Some would pass each chair going slow. They would crouch close to the row, maybe dragging their hands across the tops of each seat as they moved to the music. Hesitant to go beyond an invisible security zone, they waited in anxiety. Their faces were drawn with tension. They lingered rather than played.

Others would run and dance around the perimeter of the vacant seats. Laughing and moving by each chair quite quick, they seemed oblivious to the ticks of time. They delighted in the moment, never dwelling near a seat. They danced and pirouetted with blithe as if decorated horses and figurines, dipping and spinning on an old-fashioned calliope carousel. The children had no sense of the event to come much like the blocks of the carved wood they reminded me of.

All the others fell somewhere in between, more balanced. They enjoyed the music's rhythm and played with a passion. Although they played unfettered and had fun, they also had a strategy. They were tuned in and prepared.

It was interesting to watch each type as the game progressed. Those filled with trepidation did not smile and did not thrive in the tension and excitement. When caught without a seat, they seemed sullen and bitter. I wondered if they felt that somehow they should be guaranteed a win. They played so prepared, always close to a seat. Yet the game denied them and they were forced to leave. Did they understand they could not last forever? They denied themselves the joy of playing and were unprepared for the end. They seemed to act almost as if betrayed.

Those who were so cavalier reacted with similar hurt and anger. When the music stopped, it caught them unaware. Off balance and a distance from any chair, they pushed and shoved towards a seat. When they found it occupied, they were resentful and mean spirited. This abrupt ending marred all their fun. So whimsical at the start, they ended dejected and hostile.

Those who played with some forethought, enjoying the game but watchful, took their elimination the best. Darting toward a seat and losing, they would laugh. They had fun and *played* the game.

Some threw up their hands as if to say, "Well, I tried!"

This museful memory about a childhood game was much more. I saw it as a metaphor for life.

While at church one Sunday, I listened to our associate pastor at St. Louis DeMontfort, Father Tom Murray. His homily dealt with the reasons why things happen to us in life.

"Consider the significance of events in your lives. What do they mean?" Father Tom asked the parishioners.

Outside church after Mass, I told him the homily was poignant for me.

"I have been asking myself that very same question for two and a half years. Why did I get ALS" I rhetorically asked him. Only I had the answer.

Ever since hanging up and breaking down following the fatal phone call, I wondered why this happened to me. That first night was the longest of my life. In the darkness beyond midnight, I laid in bed unable to sleep. I felt such overwhelming vulnerability and fear. My diagnosis for a slow and agonizing death brought on by increasing paralysis was terrifying. Not a single muscle to move, no arms or hands to control, no head to turn, no voice to talk, nor tongue to swallow. In the end, no lungs to breath. Yet, all during this physical decay, I would keep a vibrant and clear intellect.

I lamented in the smothering blackness, "Oh, my Dear God! How can this be? What will I do?" I wondered aloud,

"How can I go on and face this awful future. What about my family? My children? Why did it happen?"

Through God's grace, I coped and lived beyond the statistical average for survival. I remain able to eat and take a few steps with support. I can still speak to those familiar with my voice.

More than that, I had a spiritual rebirth. Through the power of God's help, I came to think of my illness as a wonderful invitation.

He invited me, "Consider the meaning and value of your life," before the music stopped.

After diagnosis, I faced a lingering death marked by hopelessness and despair. I could have sought solace in the temporary pleasures that binges would bring. I could succumb to a hedonistic desire to 'do it all' before it is over. Credit cards could finance world travel, expensive cars, all night parties, exorbitant meals and luxurious clothing. I thought of the bumper sticker.

"He who dies with the most toys wins! Now, THAT would be some pity party!" I said to myself. God knows, that route was tempting for a while.

In the midst of this fog of fear, another vague choice began to take form. From inside, a deeper meaning for my existence and a real value in my life began to take shape. This disease could be a vehicle to true fulfillment and redemption. God willing, I was realizing this disease was not an end but the start of a new journey.

Before Amyotrophic Lateral Sclerosis struck me, I breezed through life on the outskirts of faith. I went through the perfunctory steps of my faith. I had my children baptized (my son Christopher William by Father Tom in 1985). In reality however, I was oblivious to my mortality and what lies beyond. I was certainly unprepared for the music to stop.

I lived the 'good life' of pleasures of the world, seduced by its glamour and intellect. True, I was not an evil person. Neither did I have God as the center of my life. I was kind and a good citizen. I tried it on my own terms, to be a person of character and sower of goodness. I was close, but not close enough! I was unprepared to die and face eternity.

"Chris, the music is going to stop!" God told me in specific terms.

Rather than ending the music, He gave me more time that is precious. I received a second life, one with ALS. This time was a gift beyond my worth. It brought immeasurable joy along with the pain. I experienced the profound simple pleasures of life through new eyes. I lived, learned to accept help and, in turn, help others. I have touched the lives of many through advocacy. Who would ever have dreamed I would be able to raise over eight million dollars to fight ALS?

Now reflecting on the sermon's question, 'Why did this happen and what does it mean?' has an answer. This disease is not a result. It is not an end. I believe this disease was a beginning. God, in a wisdom so perfect we can't imagine, invited me back to faith. Through His Grace, I had the strength to believe and turn away from the glitter of fool's gold. I turned toward the true light. I accepted the invitation.

There is no doubt I will live a life full of richness and happiness. It was certainly not the life I planned in my human vanity. Nevertheless, this is the life I was given. Since becoming ill, God surrounds me with countless expressions of His love. A loving family and wonderful friends encircle me. He has affirmed my life. He has shown me that I have not lived in vain.

I understand life is like a game of musical chairs. I was one of those children who danced oblivious to the impending end of music. I pranced through life unaware of my mortality. Luckily for my eternal soul, the music did not stop. God in His mercy paused the game. He gave me an undeserved chance to play again.

I rekindled my faith and found the true inner peace that The Lord provides for those who seek it. Unexplainable to some, my life has been fuller and happier than ever before. Of course, it is not without pain, sorrow and worry. These we all must have. I have fears and doubts too. My life focused as a result. Like some of the children of the musical chairs, I now have a strategy. I am finally playing the game and enjoying it too.

The healing that everyone prayed so hard for me to receive has indeed come. My soul is healthy, my spiritual health restored and I am strong. With His sustaining Grace, I shall continue. I want to live long in the shadow of Him. I am the clay and He is the potter. I am not concerned any longer about when the music will stop. He is the only one who knows for certain, so why dwell on it. Besides, there is nothing to worry about when it does stop.

The intense anxiety I had about my family lessened, as I trusted. I believe God will provide. The more I seek His strength and peace, the more He sends. We will face the trials together, with courage and faith. Held within God's arms, we shall not want.

When I consider that the music could have stopped before this invitation, I realize just how lucky I am.

Am I sick and dying? Hell No! I have just begun to live! I pray now that everyone would live realizing that the music may stop in an instant.

The lesson I learned from this was how valuable it is to get a chance to evaluate and prioritize your life. Sadly, many do not get the opportunity. I understood death could strike at any moment. I tried living life with that in mind.

The Afterglow

Rob Olson was a medium sized kid with a quizzical face, and an easy smile. He was a bit plump for a kid who was always outdoors. You could not help but notice his two large bright, white incisor teeth that dominated his round face. It made his smile infectious. Rob seemed to be a happy-go-lucky boy. He fit right in with everyone. To me, he was like any other nine-year-old. Their world was an oyster and their days spent in carefree abandon.

The screws of schooling turned snugger with advancing grades. It squeezed the carefree Rob tighter and tighter. He entered third grade fearing a continuation of his terrible cycle of failure and frustration. His parents shared the trepidation because they knew the academic demands this watershed year posed. It is the year to transition from introductions to expectation. In third grade, the work comes fast and furious. The idyllic days of a happy youngster immersed in the school tasks of reading, writing and 'rithmetic' had long since turned to a nightmare.

Rob was learning disabled.

For three years, his family clung to the hope their child would 'catch on' in time. They spent hours following assorted recommendations dutifully sent home from the school. They organized his free time, supervised his schoolwork and ran interference between teachers and their son. Both attended extra conferences. Despite the best efforts of all involved, Rob failed to prosper at learning.

He watched his peers advance to read chapter books while he still wrestled with his letters and basic words. As classmates began multiplication, he struggled to count. Letters and numbers were not familiar friends but some foreign code Rob could not decipher. No matter the exhortation, threat or bribe, the academic awakening never came. Rob was hopelessly lost in an academic world he did not understand nor did it understand him.

In the 90s, special needs education was still in its infancy. Unfortunately, for Rob and his parents, the school was ill prepared to meet his needs. Shortly after the school year began, Rob was already done. Attentiveness became indifference. Refusal replaced effort. Temper shoved aside temperance. Rob morphed into a surly, uncooperative, troublesome student at school. For the most part he sat apart, played alone and grew isolated from his schoolmates.

My gifted students were the antithesis of Robert. They were culled for their academic ability. Thus, the last place you would expect Robert to succeed was with me.

My Nature Center served the District's high potential students. Contained within the room was an amazing array of living creatures from land, sea and air. The large collection required tremendous care well beyond the time I had available. The animals needed feeding, cleaning and attention daily. I was sagging under the load even before I became ill. I could not go on without help. With the consent of my Program Supervisor and the Building Principal, I launched a special lunchtime activity in 1991, dubbed 'the Habitat Helpers' program. Students from my base school, Dickinson Avenue Elementary, volunteered their recess to work with the animals. Habitat Helpers serendipitously opened up the incredible inhabitants of the Habitat House to the entire school. At the same time, it provided the care needed to maintain the animal laboratory for my accelerated students. Because of obvious limitations of the very young, the volunteer program began, as fate would have it, with third grade.

Each group of new volunteers entered my classroom amidst chirps, croaks, cries, a squealing potbelly pig, singing bullfrogs, slithering snakes, hopping rabbits, barking prairie dog, squeaking guinea pigs, tottering tortoises, and waving lobsters as if being welcomed by the inhabitants living there. I saw each student as a helper, another set of hands, a pair of eyes and tireless young legs to shoulder my onerous load. It was a far different relationship than the traditional teacher instructing while students passively sat in stiff seats armed with a pen and paper.

Educational research clearly supports the fundamental importance of student involvement in the learning process. Habitat House taught through action. Kids worked with the animals and learned responsibility, organizational skills, math, science and language simultaneously. In the Habitat environment, Rob blended in like everyone else with one exception - he seemed to smile a bit more intensely than the others did.

Weeks ran into one another and Rob's group harmonized their tasks more efficiently than a colony of worker ants. My nature center was clean, the display cages bright and inviting but above all, the animals were well cared for and fed. The room was full of pulsating life and learning. The additional assistance provided by the Habitat Helpers offset my physical limitations.

Inevitably, Rob began to stand out. I realized there was something different about him. He had an aptitude for handling animals. He roared through his work like a freight train always asking for more things to do. He questioned everything soaking up my responses better than the clay litter that lined some of the animal cages. He stood out as an indispensable contributor to the nature center. Sure, I could see he had academic challenges, but who didn't? I was challenged myself in school. Like Rob, I struggled in school. I was disorganized, forgetful and lacked concentration in class. My high school chemistry teacher would die laughing if she could hear me today explaining the complexities of the nitrogen cycle to elementary students in a clear, understandable way by using our aquariums.

"Not bad," I could hear her say approvingly of her once struggling student. Understanding what he experienced, I used Rob's love of nature and animals to encourage him.

One afternoon Rob's parents appeared at the center. When parents showed up to talk unexpectedly, it was usually not good. Bracing for the worst, I rolled off different justification scenarios in my mind. Goodness knows Rob's parents had enough fodder to complain: soiled clothing, minor scratches, occasional animal nips and how I perennially returned the students well after recess ended. I took a deep breath, welcomed and invited them in.

They looked around, much as the children did when they first arrived. I nervously narrated a tour.

As I did, they nodded and occasionally "uh humed."

We worked our way to the rear of the room to where my desk was located. I noticed a surreptitious elbow bump accompanied by a faint smile. What was up with these two, I wondered. We finally sat down and Rob's mother, Cathy, began to talk.

I want to tell you about something that happened with Robert last night," she declared in an even, measured tone, as if she had rehearsed her lines. "I checked on Robert last night before I went to bed. I quietly opened the door of his dark room. A flashlight was on. I saw him on his bed, hunched under a tent made by covers. He glowed in the darkness. I could see him outlined there, sitting up looking down on something," she told me. I listened not knowing where this was going and how it pertained to me.

"Okay…," I replied.

Her pace quickened with anger, annoyed with his disobedience. "He went to bed an hour ago and should have been asleep."

I got the picture. Instead, he was up doing God knows what under those covers. Already convicted of an unknown infraction, she was all set to hand out justice. She was about to pounce and throw off the cover to apprehend him in the act. His mother would have reminded Robert of a snake back in Habitat House striking the food he just fed it. I waited for her to finish.

Her voice wobbled, "Do you know what I saw him doing?" Caught off guard, I had no idea what to say.

She went on before I could even answer. "He had a note-book and pencil," she confessed to me in tears. "And he, he," she stammered, "was secretly writing a letter to you in the dark using a flashlight! He wanted to tell you how happy he was and how he loved coming here."

"Really?" I tried to respond convincingly so I would appear to understand the point she was so emphatically making. I had no idea of the significance she placed on that event.

"Robbie can't write. He is dyslexic and refuses even trying anymore. Writing is torture for him," she revealed. "To get him to write something at home is not worth the battle."

Her husband clarified, "We love him and want our home to be peaceful. We have all but given up," a tinge of guilt in his voice.

"Well," I started still not fully aware of the importance she placed on it.

She interrupted, "It's this place. It's the animals. It is what you do with the kids. He WANTS to write!"

I got it. I understood. This was the kind of kid's reaction I wanted. I wanted Habitat House to create a connection between the real world and the artificial world of academics. He needed the concrete link. The animals became the teacher, the routines and tasks were the lesson plans. I was merely the facilitator. I set the stage for them to interact together. In the process, we all got what we needed.

I loved going to work.

The meeting ended with Rob's mom making the statement, "If this program has this effect on Robert, I want to do anything I can so that other children can have the same experience. I want to help you at Habitat! Can you use me?"

"Sure," I said jumping at the offer. She had no idea how much help I needed, nor how much she would ultimately give.

The mom became my volunteer assistant, gradually taking over much of the day-to-day operations for the extensive collection of animals. She was on a first name basis with Albert Einswine, our potbelly pig, Goata Meier, the pygmy goat, Balboa, an infamous eight-foot resident boa constrictor and Larry, a northern lobster. What she did not know, she learned. She coordinated scheduling other parents and the Habitat grew, flourishing with her help.

When Robert left elementary school, his younger sister, Rebecca, joined the lunchtime program. She and her mom continued Rob's legacy of hard work and commitment. We took Habitat on the road, visiting local nursing homes where the students presented their favorite animals. We established a Saturday open house so children from around the whole school district could bring their parents and enjoy the Center. More than a thousand children experienced nature up close and personal within its walls. It became well known in the community.

As Rob grew older, we had less and less contact. We ended like the bittersweet folk song, Puff the Magic Dragon. It contains the line, "Painted wings and giant rings make way for other toys," Rob grew out of Habitat. He exchanged childhood play for cars and work. Upon his high school graduation, our contact ended all together.

Not long after his graduation, I also left the Habitat when I retired from the district. In a sad development, Habitat House had to close its doors. No teacher was willing to accept the intimidating challenge of running the gifted program and maintaining Habitat House. Few colleagues shared my perspective on education or my expertise in science. The District would not hire someone to run Habitat alone. The collection was available to the community for adoption. Area nature centers accepted the remaining specimens. Interested schools took the equipment.

Although I no longer see Rob or his family and children no longer visit the Habitat, some things remain. For example, I can always see the glowing image of Cathy sitting on the bed that night. As a beacon brightly shining in the darkness of my memory, it reminds me of Puff and another magical land we called Honah-Lee.

The lesson in this was with adequate motivation set in the proper environment, young and old thrive. Diverse educational opportunity at their best over-come many barriers to authentic learning. For Rob the Habitat House was one such place.

A Master Teacher

I always thought myself a decent teacher. I loved my work and threw myself into it. For twenty-three years, I crafted my style and honed my skills. By age forty-four, I felt a seasoned and competent educator. Life, both personal and professional, had developed a rich fullness like a ripening fruit in the warmth of the summer's sun, blemishes and all. While there were some who chose superlatives to describe my work, I simply visualized myself as dedicated and hard working. There were no doubts, as actor Jack Nicholson quipped in a movie, life *was* "As good as it gets."

As good as my realm was it was also just as temporary. My world was vulnerable. My castle was built out of sand and sat beside the sea.

It all began to shift with the onset of those innocent-seeming muscle cramps. It crumbled with that call from my neurologist. It put me under a death sentence. ALS runs its nasty, fatal, paralyzing course in a flash.

The first of many choices I faced was how to spend the rest of my life. This was not a yes or no question. The answer did come easily. Quite early, I made my decision. My life was good: I wouldn't change a thing. In spite of the challenges to come, I knew I wanted to continue teaching.

Little did I realize that these darkest hours would produce my brightest moments. Along my journey with the disease. I eased from teacher to learner: from leader to explorer. The most profound lessons were still to come. As I battled ALS in the public's eye, my class, my school and my district became my allies. We all became a team, learning life's important lessons together. Here is one simple story that epitomizes the interrelationship between us all.

As mentioned, the Habitat House was an incubator producing numerous examples of this interaction. It housed many dozens of varying animal species gathered for children in a "living laboratory." Lunch periods found my room a veritable beehive of activity. Like worker drones, children were in perpetual motion tending to their charges. A large magnetic chalkboard ruled off into a grid, served as the master scheduler. It listed a myriad of feeding details including animal names, cage numbers, food types and amounts.

The chalkboard was a self-directing manager. Each animal had a small square magnet occupying the last square of the grid. One side was red and green on the other. When a student scanned the board for a task to complete, they saw which jobs needed to be completed -they were green. Upon selection of a particular "green, go" job, the student must turn the magnet to red, signaling, to other children, "Stop—it's done." Then they set about doing the task. Perhaps they needed to weigh out twenty-one grams of oats for the Egyptian spiny mouse, change the hay in the Pigmy goat enclosure, measure 125 milliliters of water for the chinchilla or sample the Ph in one of the aquariums. Each new marking period, another crop of lunchtime would-be naturalists stride into Habitat, ready for work.

On one of the orientation sessions for a new group, a timid third grader listened to my detailed procedures. When instructed, she approached the board and viewed her options. Her head rotated as she scanned the list. After an inordinate interval, she turned and stared off in my direction. Sensing something, I labored toward her.

"Mr. P, I need help. I want to feed the iguana but can't," I barely heard her say over the busy background noise.

I bent down to inquire the nature of her problem. I gently probed, "Do you understand the board?"

Her head bobbed in affirmation. Perplexed, I searched wider. "And, you know where the supplies are?"

Again, she nodded. Her eyes, on level with mine, seemed tense and unsure. I remained hunched to be close. Her statement stumped me. "Well honey, what is it?"

She raised her hand, index finger extended and pointed to the chalkboard. Her arm angled up and fixed on the iguana. It was the highest choice.

"It's too high; I can't reach to turn the magnet. My arms are too short; will you do it for me?"

The pint-sized waif stood looking at me awaiting my intervention. I froze, helpless, as I sensed my own paralyzed arms hanging limply at my side. I, the teacher, was unable to help this young girl with her simple request. She waited with an innocent stare that burned through me. I interpreted her body language as saying, *"Well, are you going to help me or not?"* I couldn't.

As I faced the decision to teach with increasing disabilities brought on by ALS, a haunting thought always shadowed me. Would I recognize when the time comes that I should retire, when my limitations exceed my contributions? Sixty odd years ago, my disease's namesake, Lou Gehrig, faced the same decisive moment. After a historic string of over 2,000 games stretching 13 years, Lou left baseball.

"Leave at the top of your game" is a mantra spoken by all challenged with a declining performance. I wrestled with that idea as I faced this young girl. I felt on the cusp of where I reached the point when I was at the top with the decline ahead. I couldn't help her with the simplest routine request. Worse, my ALS interfered with her progress. I was hurting rather than helping.

Without intending, this sweet, eager, young child taught me a lesson in life and about myself.

ALS was the curriculum and I became the learner.

In my intellect, I knew real teaching was a magical interaction between teacher and learner. John Dewey, the father of American education, captured it

He told us, "Learning is not a spectator sport."

You learn best through involvement in real problem solving. In spite of this, I was a prisoner of the teacher's need to "always know and to be in charge."

Like a blacksmith's anvil, ALS reshaped my life. It forged me anew, stretching who and what I was. This young girl was doing the same thing. I was learning that there are times we are not the ones to solve things by ourselves.

I wracked my brain to come up with a resolution to her quandary. I failed to see a solution. With a gentle honesty, I asked her a question.

"Are you aware of my muscle disease?"

She fidgeted a smiled and whispered, "Yes."

"Well hon, I can't help you. My arms are too weak. I can't raise them up that far."

Relieved at my own truthfulness, I awaited a response. I anticipated her to make a new selection of a different animal, one that was more within her reach instead. However, she continued to look at me. Her mind was fixed. She wanted the iguana. Retreat was not an option she entertained.

In a flash, it came to me. "Hon, I can't solve your problem alone. But, if we work as a team, I think we can solve it together."

She looked puzzled.

"Well," I continued, "your arms are too short, my arms are too weak. However, if we work together and help each other, we can do it."

"Okay," she waited for more.

"I will give you the length of my arms and you give me the strength of yours."

I motioned to her to grasp my thin, limp arm hanging uselessly at my side. Recognizing the unorthodoxy of it all, she hesitated before taking my arm.

"Great," I exclaimed and encouraged her to lift and to push it higher.

Stretching on her tippy toes and strained with the deadweight of my long arm. She inched my hand close to the top of the chalkboard, a good six feet high. Her fingers pressed into the flesh of my upper arm and I heard a moan as she made a last effort. Hitting the magnet, my fingers fumbled and managed to flip it to red. Spent, she let my arm go. It fell and thudded against my leg. Then she bounded off, content to do her job. With her back to me she shouted, "Thanks." It was but a brief moment and it was over.

I stood there. The impact of what happened slowly sunk in. I realized I was no longer 'able' in a physical sense. I learned from ALS that I was no longer in charge of circumstance. The girl taught me that I alone was not always the solution.

ALS had branded limitations into me. Experience did the same with potential.

I realized also, we must be a team. A true team united by common goals and purpose. Strength should be measured in our collective strengths and not by our individual weakness.

It took me awhile to get Dewey's words. Twenty-five years to be exact. Guess I am a slow learner. Better late than never.

I continued to teach in the classroom for another eight years. My muscle deterioration advanced. I experienced the pain of growing more aware of everything I could no longer do. At the same time, I rejoiced as I considered all I can do. I've learned: spirit and determination combined with teamwork are limitless.

Each day brings a new challenge. It also brings an opportunity to learn and grow. ALS, rather than a death sentence, has become the real master teacher. It teaches my family, friends and me.

There were some who chose superlatives to describe my teaching. I know the real Master Teacher.

The lesson in this was teamwork produces results beyond individual's abilities separately. We must measure our ability not by our individual weaknesses but by the collective strength we have alongside others united for a common goal.

Two Visitors

I enjoy writing poetry, especially free verse. It allows me the freedom to conjure up images, emotions and scenes without the demands and limits of prose. A poem gives me the opportunity to take the reader on quantum leaps of thought as I tell my story. For me, it is a powerful medium to express my complicated feelings and ideas. It is a rich, fertile field to plant them. I wrote this a year after my diagnosis.

I have for so long, loved the ocean.
I often went to its shore.
It seemed to just beckon me
with its carpet of soft sand and cool, blue water.

I can recall so very well the scent of sweet,
salted air that greeted me each time I neared.
In my mind's eye, I still see its pallets of pebbles:
a rainbow of hues cast along the water's edge.
I remember those long and winding wind-tossed
lines of shells, seaweed and bone
twisted down the shoreline

In it I found a treasure chest of nature's surprises;

there were mermaid's purses, jingle shells, feathers, shiny
crab backs and small,
colorfully polished glass chips.

mm, and I recall too,
the melodies murmured by the gentle surf.

Of all of these images however,
I remember most the peace.
I found there an abiding air of harmony.
I sensed contentment, a joy.
Serenity

Once while there, a violent storm blew in.
As I watched, the distant skies grew dark and ominous:
the blue blotted by blackness,
the light breeze was whipped to a wind.
The sweet, salted air turned acrid and accosted me.
It beat against my unprotected face. The pebbles stung as
they pelted me,
raging out of control as if as angry as the wicked wind that
flung them.

And the gentle, murmuring surf?

It wailed eerily, hurling itself up and onto the beach.
It mouthed a moan, dragging itself back,
scraping across the sand
and into the jaws of the next frothing wave.
My gentle ocean and its soothing shore

turned cruel and unkind:
unfit for me or any living thing.
A sanctuary destroyed, it had morphed
into a bellowing beast.
The sands seemed to shift under my feet.
Uneasy, I began to retreat,
reluctantly yielding my paradise.

At that moment, in the height of this fury,
out of the darkened heavens
dropped a solitary, soaring gull.

Spellbound, I watched it being buffeted
by the turbulence.
To my amazement it held fast.
With wings bent awkwardly
and feathers twisted awry,
it struggled to ride the shearing winds,
unwilling to be beaten back.
As if defiantly claiming its right to the beach,
to this paradise,
it stubbornly hovered right above me.
I thought, how triumphant this new visitor.
A contrast to the unwanted and ill-tempered other one.
In my soul, I sensed the gull balanced the storm.
They seemed to equal each other in strength and intensity.

Slowly, I felt the serenity raise within me once more.

So steeled, I too, stayed.

We silently rode out the storm together.
After a time together we parted.
Distanced by lives and nature
but none the less woven into an unseen web,
we were one that gull and I.

Once, while busy living, another storm blew in.
Shrouded in stealth, ALS closed in.
It too was also terribly turbulent.
There were times when it was all I could do
to just hang on.
A vicious and unwanted vortex swirled about me.
Things slammed in from all directions, like the pebbles of
the first storm.

I was pelted. I was stung.
I was being beaten down. My stance tilted
as the earth moved under my feet.
Again I was being forced to yield.
I was so small and this was so big.
Like a hurricane, ALS was knocking me down
and sweeping me away.
I was afraid once more.

Then someone simply took a moment, to just "fly by."
Maybe it was to only say hello,
perhaps lend a helping hand

or to let me know that they were still there.

So unexpected but dear God, so welcomed.
It was you. How did you know? Did you even realize?

Do you see? You were my gull,
forever soaring right overhead.
Your presence renewed my strength
and rekindled my wonder.

Distanced by lives and by nature, certainly unplanned, we
were also woven into a web of life.

Know this my friend: we can weather the storm,
hold fast to our beach
and maintain that abiding peace.
But then we too must part.

May God always bless you
by sending you His gulls during your storm.

In 1970, the first year I taught, one of my students, Danny
Conroy had surgery requiring a long convalescence. I became
his home tutor and went to his house daily after school. I
grew close to his entire family including five siblings. Twenty
years later, the district hired one of his younger sisters as an
elementary teacher. She was assigned to Dickinson Avenue.
Jeannette was an active, environmentally focused teacher
making frequent outdoor trips with her class. She often went
to the beach and brought back specimens for my classroom's

numerous salt-water aquariums in Habitat House. We chatted many times about the marine environment. We shared a deep love of children and the sea. One day, standing outside the door of my room chatting, I launched into an extemporaneous ocean poem. It evolved into this poem. I dedicate it to Jeannette and her family.

The lesson in this was it may only take a simple 'Hello, how are you today?' to make a difference to people barely hanging on. Be proactive and reach out to someone. They may need it beyond your understanding.

Dying to Dive

As summer neared its end in 2018, my wife and I wanted to get in one more fun activity with our 11-year-old grandson, Patrick. Since he and I are both avid anglers and nature lovers, she made a suggestion tying both together.

"Let's go to the aquarium," she said.

We visited the shark tank, fed stingrays and marveled at the butterfly exhibit. Then we came upon the large, brightly lit, open reef display. I sat in front of the huge thick glass, hypnotized by the reef's gloriousness. Bittersweet memories of my tropical diving days came flooding through. The last time I dove was in 1997, four years after my ALS diagnosis.

At the time of that dive, Christopher, my son, was 12 years old, the age youngsters can qualify for a junior diving certificate. For my son's January birthday, I surprised him with scuba diving lessons. Over the winter, I took him to classes to qualify for his certificate. He was the only child in the group geared for adults and managed to pass the written exam. Then, he followed up with an open water test and received his certification in the summer. He was ready.

As a father and a diver, I desperately wanted to share that world with him before that happened. Now with his certification, it was within reach. The undersea world is like visiting a different planet. It is an alien world, a place where we are only

51

visitors. There, life is so fundamentally different. Shapes and colors are as remarkable as they are unreal.

I began exploring options for a trip. I chose St. John in the Virgin Islands. It had a national park where we could camp, and a world famous water environment. Because of my paralyzed arms and hands, along with weak legs—combined with Christopher's age—I expected to have a difficult time getting a dive shop to accommodate us. I called a few local scuba shops explaining my physical condition and they declined my request. Growing worried my calls took a more frenetic urgency.

Out of the phone came, "Hello."

I opened with, "I know this will sound crazy, but please hear me out. I am dying from Lou Gehrig's disease and I want to take my 12-year-old diving before I die. My arms are already paralyzed but I still can swim well under water." I continued before he could respond negatively. "He is all set. I took him for his certificate. He has his open water dive completed. He is a good swimmer and mature for his age." I wrapped up with, "I understand my request is unusual and will be a headache. It means the world to me for a chance to dive with my son. I need you to help make the dream a reality. Please work with me."

After listening, the owner replied, "Mr. Pendergast, if you want to dive that badly, we'll do whatever it takes so you get to dive with your boy! Come down and we'll make it work."

"Oh, thank you for this chance. You made my summer. I can't wait." I shot back.

Over the Jewish Holy Days in September when school closed, we headed to the Virgin Islands. As my wife watched us trudge off towards the plane dragging our luggage, with my son doing most of the work, she wondered out-loud, "What did I just do?" The sight of us actually leaving made it real. "I sent a paralyzed man off on a diving trip out of the country accompanied only by a twelve-year-old child!"

"How are you doing?" I asked him.

"Okay, Dad. Let's go or we will miss the plane." He looked back to hurry me as we walked towards the gate

We headed for an adventure of a lifetime. I had no idea it would be an epic experience-a forever memory.

The harbor resembled a sheet cake covered with blue frosting. Humid, sweet, salted air filled our nostrils walking down the long wharf. We boarded a specialized dive vessel designed for the open water reef diving along with several other people. All eyes were on us as my son assisted me aboard, while trying to lug our gear at the same time. The boat headed out of the harbor towards the reefs that form a protective ring around the Island.

The ocean swells caused us to rock and roll. In unison to their rhythm, I staggered like a drunken sailor. Christopher lurched to hold me up each time I weaved towards the railing. We must have looked like a pair of amateur comics rehearsing for a talent show. The engines eventually quieted and the captain dropped anchor just beyond the sensitive coral to prevent damaging it.

Getting me suited up was a challenge. With several dive assistants helping, I struggled but managed to get the skintight wet suit on. However, the all-important weight belt proved to be impossible. We were unable to cinch the thirty pounds of lead around my waist. With no weight, I would float like a cork because of the buoyant suit and the one hundred cubic feet of compressed air in the tank strapped to my back. Faced with failure, the Dive Master proposed a solution violating all the rules.

"Instead of wearing the weights on a belt, we can put them in the pockets of your buoyancy compensator vest. You won't be able to shed them easily by releasing the buckle in an emergency, but it will get you weighted."

Weighted down I was able to dive. If I needed to surface immediately in a dire emergency, I couldn't. The weights would be stuck in my pockets and I would drown. In a normal situation, this would never be an option. Given my circumstance, there was no alternative. Either I chose to dive with this added danger or I sat on the boat. My son's eyes implored me as I realized there was no choice.

"Let's do it," I said.

Experienced divers get a dive master to supervise a group. In our case, my son got his own "buddy" and a separate one went with me. He wanted to be at my side to protect me from common problems that would be life threatening for me, like a dislodged mask or dropped mouthpiece. He also could adjust my buoyancy compensator so I wouldn't sink or float, remaining neutral in the water. Christopher entered the water with the traditional backflip from the side rail of the boat while I stepped off the rear swim platform. Our adventure began.

Once in the water, we descended a steep coral wall not unlike a cliff you encounter when hiking in the mountains. The face of the reef dropped off and we swam nearly vertical as we went down. Every 15 or 20 feet there was a complete change in environments because of diminishing light penetration.

Each new zone brought more fantastic delights than the previous one. Different corals dazzlingly displayed their varied shapes, textures and colors. Teals, turquoise, magentas, marigolds, pinks, purples, emeralds and of course, azures flooded our eyes. The schools of fish changed as well. Tropical fish are riots of color with improbable combinations and fantastical bodies. There were moving clouds of stripes, dancing polka dots, and other stunning designs swimming past. Their names conjure imaginations in land lovers who never get to see them in their natural habitat: Parrot, Angel, Trigger, Zebra, Convict, Lion or Clown, for examples. These fish are more majestic and beautiful than the names suggest.

Life teemed everywhere. Gelatinous anemone arms of every length, color and width waved in unison moved by an unheard melody. It reminded me of human arms swaying together at a rock concert or a wave at a football game. Black pincushions punctuated the lines of coral, as the sea urchins were everywhere. Darkened crevices hid mysterious, reclusive creatures—an octopus tentacle or lobster antennae revealing its occupants. Sea stars of all hues confirmed the reef was heaven on earth, or more accurately, under it.

Once we reached the bottom at about 60 feet, the maximum we could go without decompressing, I rested on the sugar sand sea floor. I rolled onto my back and in the total silence of the moment, I stared at the heavens far above. It felt like I was in a vestibule of a medieval cathedral looking up at a huge stained glass window. Shafts of light pierced the water, filtered downward and reflected off the reef's rainbow of colors, creating a massive fresco. And there, in front of God's masterpiece, was my son moving slow with the rhythm of the ocean. I filled with rapture. As joyous as I was, there was more to come!

A short swim away from the base of the reef was a trough that dropped an additional 30 or 40 feet. The Dive Master accompanying us signaled to go deeper. I declined, opting to watch and allow my son to experience the deeper dive solo. How many kids this age have been almost a hundred feet under the ocean alone! Because of the additional depth, they could only dive down a moment and immediately return to the shallower depth at the bottom of the reef. As the pair tilted down and dove, I moved over them. I watched my son grow small. His fluid movements entranced me.

I moved directly over him and stared at the bubbles coming out of his regulator. They were literally the breaths of his life. The large bubbles floated upward, breaking into multiple orbs as they rose through the water. I positioned myself to allow the bubbles to hit me. As they did, they burst into hundreds of small ones. The tiny bubbles stuck to my black wetsuit and covered me from mask to flipper, similar to a glass of sparkling champagne! The light shined through the bubbles causing them to shimmer. My black wetsuit sparkled like countless miniature diamonds. His breath of life encased me. I bobbed on the breath of my son, my offspring, the flesh of my flesh. I experienced a Oneness. It was surreal, never to be forgotten.

I never dove again. What a way to end 30 years of diving.

My wife and Patrick already moved on to other exhibits.

As I left, I mumbled, "Will Patrick ever dive? I hope so."

The lesson in this is you are never too young, old or sick to enjoy new, memorable adventures. Do not let such opportunities slip by.

A Rewarding Award

Our son was an avid athlete who loved scholastic sports. Each season offered a sport he enjoyed. While in eighth grade in '99, he played on the soccer team in the fall, the middle school basketball team in the winter and their baseball team in the spring. I guess he inherited my wife's genes for sport. She was also an athlete in school and was a successful physical education teacher and coach.

We beamed with joy as he proudly announced he was receiving a sports award at the annual Award Assembly. "Can you guys come to see it?"

"I have an engagement I cannot not break," my wife told him. He was disappointed that she could not go.

"You are coming right Dad?"

"I would not miss it, Buddy. I can't wait!" We all looked forward to his recognition for athletic achievements.

The day turned into a fiasco. It involved a simple, basic human function done every day. For ALS patients, nothing is simple.

For readers over forty, Ted Koppel, the anchor on the late evening news program, Nightline, was a well-known figure. Scoring an interview on the show guaranteed a national audience. Brandies University Sociology Professor, Morrie Schwartz, of *Tuesdays with Morrie* fame, appeared twice on the show. The first time was in March of 1995. He shared his experience living and dying with ALS. My recent inclusion into the exclusive ALS club made me an intense observer. With every new sentence Morrie delivered, came another unsettling realization about my own future path.

Terminally ill patients choosing death had become a national fixation. Euthanasia was a hot topic. Mike Wallace brought this to the public in a controversial show aired on 60 Minutes. He showed an ALS patient euthanized on camera. Since the early 90s, Dr. Kevorkian was assisting people die who face catastrophic illness, such as ALS.

The host wanted his audience to understand the totality of the disease. Koppel asked Morrie, "Can you describe what living with ALS is like?"

Morrie told of his progression, trials coping and struggle accepting help.

Koppel prompted Schwartz to retell some of their off camera discussions about loss of function and independence. Specifically, he wanted Morrie to relate the signal that he had enough of enduring the progressive paralysis. In a bold move Koppel queried, "Please share with the audience when you will know you don't want to live anymore."

Koppel asked him to use the crude example made earlier off camera. The lens panned to a close-up of Schwartz' face. It appeared quizzical. He replied, "I don't know if I can say this on television."

The tough veteran reporter encouraged Morrie to be honest, "Go ahead, say it on TV because in many respects it brings it home (the devastation of the disease) much better than anything else." My heart froze.

"Well," Morrie chose his words carefully, "I will know I've had enough when I can no longer wipe my own ass." That is when Morrie would end his life. He then waxed philosophical, lamenting about growing dependence and declining quality of life.

As a patient facing the loss of walking, eating, talking and breathing, his reference to a trite subject like toileting surprised me. God, what a relatively insignificant thing to hang a decision to live or die on. Out of all one can lose, how could he include *that* to signal the end of the line?

When most people awake in the morning they ask ordinary questions such as, "What is the weather? What should I wear?" I was not ordinary. I was an ALS patient struggling to continue to work.

I had to ask, "Will I need to go to the bathroom in the next 8 hours?"

Because of my paralysis, I no longer was able to independently toilet. Female colleagues surround me in an elementary school. There were few options available if I had to use the bathroom at work. This reality framed my workday.

The morning of the ceremony, my son arose excited for the day to begin. It was hard for him to wait for the event. Affirming the specialness of the occasion, I said, "Buddy, I am really proud of you and I am looking forward to watching you get your award."

"I'm leaving," Christine shouted as she grabbed her lunch.

"Bye mom!" Christopher yelled back before running out the door himself.

"See you guys. Love you." I added. My ride was running late. It was 7:00 a.m.

59

Around nine o'clock, in the middle of a lesson at school, I felt an uneasy rumbling in my belly. This was not a good sign. By lunchtime, the sensations were steady along with an occasional cramp. I studied the clock calculating the remaining time and strategizing how to make it through until I got home. At the end of the day, I zipped on my scooter toward the parking lot where I would rendezvous with a volunteer driver for the one-hour trip home.

I short-changed my car pool driver on conversation during the ride as I concentrated on holding on and holding it in a little longer. My pride shouted to maintain pleasantries but my insides screamed otherwise.

Summoning up the courage and the words, I delicately explained, "I'm sorry but I gotta get home as soon as possible. I need to have a bowel movement. Please step on it!"

"Sure! I will get you there, don't worry," as they sped towards my house.

I promised, "Otherwise it would not be pretty if I didn't."

The car did not even come to a stop in the driveway and I moved to exit. My driving companion raced around to help raise me up from the low car seat. Although my arms no longer functioned, I had enough strength in my legs to walk short distances (my friends and family referred to it as stagger). Like a miracle out of Lourdes, I found the power to dash to the door. My driver threw it open for me and I headed for the bathroom upstairs in my room. On good days, the thirteen stairs were a marathon climb for me. That day they loomed before me as an Ironman Triathlon course. I gave it my best attempt.

Several steps up, my luck ran out. So did my bowels. Anger filled me as I failed so close to success. Even though I lost control, I had no choice but to go on. I continued to go up as well as out. Each remaining step was a torturous, slow journey. By the time I reached the toilet, I was soiled and there was a total mess behind me. I was disgusted...

I collapsed down on the seat. My paralysis made removing my fouled clothes impossible. Unable to clean myself either, upset and dejected, I sat resigned to staying there until my wife came home. Sitting on the toilet for a couple of hours was not the worst fate in the world. I could have fallen, lying on the floor, in pain. I totally forgot about the award assembly until I heard the door close downstairs.

"Dad, are you ready?" my son's voice lofted up from the foyer.

"Holy crap, now what am I gonna do?"

Throughout my disease, I attempted to keep my life as normal and routine as possible. I refused to have my children's memories of our life etched by illness. I did whatever I could to be ordinary. I did not hide my disease nor its outcome, but neither did I let it define us. I strived to avoid making my problems my children's problems.

When my son ran up the stairs to check on me, he found my trail. His voice sounded edgy as he called "Oh man! What happened? Dad, are you alright?"

I managed to slam the bathroom door with my foot before calling out.

"Buddy, I had an accident. I am a mess in here. Stay out," I commanded. "I went all over myself. My clothes are disgusting. I don't want you to come in," I shouted from behind the door.

He protested, "But Dad, I have my assembly today!"

"I know Bud," my voice thick, "but, there's nothing I can do. I'm sorry."

"I'll help you. Let me come in," he implored.

My mind swirled with conflicting feelings. My dignity, my pride, my fatherhood, they all told me to tough it out and wait for my wife.

"No, Bud, I am gonna wait for Mom," I did not realize how he was feeling.

"Please, I want to help you!" he insistently continued. "Please, Daddy."

My heart broke as I stood my ground.

"Buddy, I am OK. I just have to wait for Mom."

I wanted to spare him the unpleasantness. I wanted to avoid creating a memory of this distasteful task he was so ardently requesting to perform. It was my job to be stoic and deal with this alone, I told myself. Somehow, I thought by taking this stance, I regained some control over my illness. My decision to keep him out allowed me to retain a remnant of my former self. I was not letting ALS rule my life.

Pride distorted my thinking.

"But, I *want* you to come to the assembly," he emphatically proclaimed.

"Buddy, you'll have to go by yourself. What can I do?" my voice rose an octave as I shouted back through the door.

"I will clean you. It's okay. I want to help you. Please, Daddy."

His voice had a tone that sliced right through the wooden divider. I did not want him to have to see me like this. No young boy should need to wipe fecal-filled folds on his father's body. It just wasn't right.

It is also not right that a father doesn't accompany his son to an award ceremony.

I was living the moment Morrie Schwarz spoke about to Ted Koppel. This was the great chasm he chose to separate life and death. Morrie wanted to die before he had to endure the indignity of someone wiping his ass.

The tiny bathroom shrunk as I sat there thinking. His pleadings became background noise as I wrestled with myself. Was I really protecting him? Or, was it my hidden pride? Did my decision benefit him or was I punishing him?

He pulled me back to the present with his crackling.

"Daddy?"

I made a pivotal decision, one, which helped me understand more about the essence of fatherhood. It's about what he needs and wants, not my wishes. I should be at his ceremony, not wallowing in my own inabilities, stubbornly refusing his offer of help.

"Ok, Buddy. Come on in."

With grace and maturity far beyond his age, he got me ready. We spent the next forty-five minutes cleaning the room and me. Tension yielded to comedy as we exchanged various bathroom humors over the situation. Rather than being horrible and embarrassing, it resulted in a spiritually growing and bonding experience.

With minutes to spare, he had me in my power wheel chair and we set off for the school a few blocks away. He had me looking like a million bucks.

We rolled into a jammed gymnasium, which doubled as the auditorium for the school. Squirming middle schoolers packed the bleachers. Folding chairs, separated by narrow rows filled the floor.

"I have to sit with the kids," I tilted my head trying to point to the rows of designated chairs. Christopher left to sit near the stage. I negotiated the tight path toward the parents sitting area.

The award ceremony was a cookie cutter program similar to countless others. Kids cheered and parents clapped with each presentation. I too hooted and clapped hearing Buddy's name. He won an award for playing three seasons, a difficult achievement. My chest swelled and my face glowed as he approached the podium. For an instant, his eyes searched the crowd. I saw a broad grin grow on his lips when he spotted me. I grinned right back, so grateful he persevered to get me here.

The Principal concluded the ceremony by presenting the prestigious Triple C Award sponsored by the New York State Attorney General's office.

"This is a special recognition given to students nominated by schools because they epitomize character, commitment and courage. Our school is proud to have an awardee this year," the principal told the audience.

Then, he described the fine qualities of the student selected to receive the award. Listening, I could not help but admire the unknown youngster.

"He must be quite a kid," I said aloud.

The Principal's voice rose to dramatize the moment. The name echoed across the room.

"Buddy Pendergast," reverberated, followed by a thunderous applause. Some teachers stood up leading to a standing ovation from everyone. The room rocked.

"Mr. Pendergast, please come up to the stage to be with your son as he receives the award."

I made my way to the podium. Joyfully, I sat at his side and watched him accept. I looked out at the approving crowd and reflected on the events, a short time ago which got us here. They would never know the true depth of character and courage exhibited by my son. They thought they knew my son's story based on TV and newspaper coverage of his role on the two ALS Ride for Life trips. They saw him bicycling and skating to Washington alongside my power wheelchair. Those snippets merely pierced the surface of his character.

Barely an hour ago, he was able to convince his reluctant father to accept the unacceptable. They should have seen him scrub the soiled rug, remove my dirty clothes, and wipe the excrement from my skin. He volunteered to do it with happiness. He did it simply to have his dad be with him.

Now, he was up on stage. What a sweet and unpredictable world…

It would be difficult to imagine a more deserving youngster that afternoon. When Christopher stuck out his hand to shake with the Principal, I wept openly.

I nearly missed one of the proudest moments of my life. Thank God, I ignored the suggestion Morrie made.

The lesson in this was adversity builds character. My son had a difficult childhood marked by losing his normal Dad. Instead, he lived with a dependent, dying one. He grew immeasurably, but bore a heavy price. He developed patience, wisdom and empathy beyond his years. Bad things can produce good results.

On Angels Wings

Like a bright porch light on a summer's eve drawing moths, the Galapagos Islands attract nature lovers from all over. They were the enchanted islands filled with magical animals. Ever since I was first aware of them, I wanted to go. Living got in the way and like most, I focused on building a career and raising a family. There was little time and less money for such exotic dreams. The idea of visiting them slipped to a distant recess in my mind.

Of course, the ALS erased my family's normal game plan. We implemented a new one that accounted for my assumed calendar reduction. Living in the moment and not putting things off became less an abstraction and more real in my daily life. As the reality of my disease sunk in, I wanted to make sure our family would have no regrets about lost opportunities. In 1995 we held a family meeting. We discussed what everyone wanted to do as a special family trip.

Christine said, "Ireland." So in 1996, when I was still able to walk well, we flew to the Emerald Isle. Refusing to go on canned tours, we rented a car, bought maps and set out to explore our ancestral homeland. The smaller the road the better to get off the beaten path. My wife wanted to drive because she thought it was safer. Before we left the airport's rental car lot, she managed to bang the side view mirror driving too close on the left side of the road. I offered to drive but was overruled. The trip was wonderful.

My daughter, "California." Melissa and I flew to the West Coast and Hollywood in 1998. We toured Beverly Hills and she drove me in a rented convertible through the fabled canyons on Rodeo Drive past the mansions of Hollywood's elite. She and I strolled along famed Muscle Beach where she tried to walk a few steps ahead of me gawking at tanned, trim hunks. We had a ball.

Christopher wanted, "Magic Kingdom." He got to go to a 'magic kingdom' but not one created by Walt Disney. In a few years he and I would go to the real deal.

"I want to go to the Galapagos;" I announced.

My choice came as no surprise to Christine. One of our first dates was fishing. I always shared my love of science and nature with my family. I dragged my daughter on all of my classroom field trips. By the time she was a young teen, she pretty much had her full of muddy marshes, flowered fields and blazing beaches. Then 21 and in college, she preferred music, sports and boys. My son, on the other hand, 8 years her junior, was still enthralled by the magic of nature.

My wife had obligations at home and was not interested. Melissa outgrew her nature days. I made the decision. I was taking my 14-year-old son to Ecuador. It did not enter my mind I was physically impaired: unable to dress myself, hold my own passport or take care of him. I guess my excitement blurred my reasoning.

"Hey Buddy, do you want to go to Galapagos with me?"

When I asked he lit up, "Really Dad, are you kidding with me?"

"Yes, I'm being serious."

"Sure, that would be awesome," he said oblivious also to the ramifications of going alone with me.

Under normal circumstances taking a child to a third world country by yourself would be dicey. Considering the totality of my needs, plus the location half way around the world, my plan was almost over the edge of reason. In my situation, I thought why not? Foolishly, I ignored all the potential problems that could occur.

A local travel agency specializing in adventure vacations suggested, "Start with a three-day stay in Ecuador's capitol city of Quito. Then take a bus to the coastal city of Guayaquil and catch a short flight over the ocean to the Island's only airport on San Cristobal."

"Once on the island we travel on a small cruise ship and island hop. It's going to be awesome," I told everyone.

It was an exhausting and full schedule for the able-bodied. Clearly, we had challenges ahead. My wife recalls leaving us at JFK airport in New York City. She watched her young son weighed down by travel bags, identification carriers, and my money-filled wallet disappear at an airport into a sea of people. I tagged along at his side. Reversing roles, she entrusted my care to our child in a foreign speaking country more than five thousand miles away.

"My God, what have I just done?" she found herself saying.

At the end of a six-hour-flight, we arrived over the capitol tucked in between the mountains. After viewing expanses of mountainous wilderness through the tiny window, the urban center suddenly appeared revealing the airport in the valley I could not believe we would land there. Airbrakes hammered us back in our seat as the speeding jet attempted to slow on the short runway. The pilot put us down as easily as pulling into a driveway.

Christopher handled himself admirably when we gathered our luggage and passed through the airport security. I was the mouth and he was the hands.

"We make a great team Buddy," I told him. "You make me proud, son." I ached to pat him on the back. When asked if ALS is painful, I think of moments like this.

The hotel was not a far drive. It was enough to show the third-world poverty that gripped the city. Reliable electric service was something most inhabitants did without. Each day rolling blackouts moved from one neighborhood to another. The government could not produce enough electricity to meet the demand of its one million residents. Our hotel catered to the growing tourist trade and had its own generators to produce continuous electricity.

We watched men washing their taxicabs in the public fountains alongside woman and children washing clothes. These experiences were our first introductions to the reality of Ecuadorian life. Christopher and I would have many more. For now, we were safe and comfortable at the hotel. Tomorrow was another day.

The concierge arranged side trips appropriate for my limitations. We toured the historic heart of Quito from which Spain once ruled her New World Empire. It was another world walking among the buildings of the UNESCO Heritage site of the Monastery of San Francisco, built in the 1550s.

Visiting an authentic indigenous people's open market gave us a unique flavor for life outside the urban, civilized city center. An estimated 20% of Ecuador's population is indigenous, the largest of any South American country.

"Are you ready to see the other Ecuador, Christopher?" as we prepared to board a public bus bound for a village about 20 miles outside the city.

Besides a purple haired, pierced and tattooed young free-spirited girl, we were the only Americans on the packed bus. Christopher's eyes were glued to the window in disbelief as we passed deplorable hovels people called homes. I fixed my eyes out the front windshield at the thin corkscrew ahead, which passed as a road. Our driver casually took the hairpin turns that would make a Colorado driver cautious. The intimidating bus forced other vehicles to the side on the narrow, twisted roadway.

The shanty suburbs of Quito finally gave way to forests and fields nestled in valleys. We entered a regional village, which served as a centralized location where farmers brought their produce. We departed the bus just beyond the congested central square.

"Stay close, and hold my hand." I told him.

Indigenous people in native dress roamed everywhere. Standard issue were colorful ponchos all made locally by hand from llama wool. Many of the people wore crisp white linen shirts and slacks.

"How would you like to live here Bud? Did you notice the men are sewing? The women are doing the farm work." I asked.

In the reversal of American roles, male members of this tribe were the tailors and made all of the clothing. Women toiled in the fields and tended the animals. Everyone wore broad brimmed straw hats.

The market took up the entire town square, probably a couple of acres. Being a suburban boy, I was familiar with county fairs and fairways jammed with vendors. It reminded me of a large flea market. Sellers displayed fifty or a hundred-pound gunnysacks stacked around some wood propped on a pile of other sacks. There were endless varieties of beans, corn and other grains. Many of the seeds were completely new. Other vendors had fruit, most of which I also did not recognize. There were vegetables everywhere, especially tomatoes and root crops such as potatoes or yams. Every size, color and shape were available.

"Eeww, that's gross." Christopher said. As we neared the meat and fish vendors, I saw what he meant.

"Oh yeah, I see what you're talking about." The sight was disturbing.

Entire carcasses laid out in the baking midday sun. Customers picked out a piece of meat that was summarily sliced then wrapped the selection in newspaper. Local fish, fowl and mammal hung from overhead racks. Flies were everywhere so thick and persistent they were not even shooed away.

"How they don't get sick I'll never know." I said to my son. "I feel sick looking at it."

He spied a moving sack under one table. He heard unmistakable yelping of puppies. His hand tightened on my arm, pulling me down to his level.

"Daddy, what's in there?" he nervously asked. He already knew the answer but wanted to be told something different.

"I guess they are puppies," I answered honestly.

"Why are they in the bag?" he asked.

"These people are very poor and meat is very expensive," I told him, trying to anticipate his reaction. "So, sometimes they have to eat things that we would not."

"Yea, but they are only puppies," he said, "How can they do that?"

"They have no choice. It is that or go hungry." He rejected my answer, pulling my arm away as he turned to leave with tears in his eyes. I am not sure whom he was crying for, the puppies, or the people. Perhaps both.

Beside the produce and meat for sale, there were a host of other commodities and native crafts. Wool, fabrics and clothes were everywhere. Many artisans worked with clay, making every item the village needed. Row after row of finished pieces dried in the equatorial sun. Because it was Christmas, there were religious statues and figurines all over the place.

"Hey dad I like that one a lot," pointing to a Star of Bethlehem shining over a small hacienda.

"Okay, tell the man," I told him, "now we barter to reach a price." We talked through gestures and money pointing.

"Why are you trying to lower the price? They need the money Daddy." He said.

I explained about the traditional ritual of arriving at a fair price. When satisfied with our offer, the artist wrapped it up and handed it to me. I could not carry it. I motioned with my head and body for him to give it to my son.

"I'll take it," he said to the confused seller. Christopher smiled and grabbed the package.

We walked back toward the bus, gabbing and gawking. I heard a crash. I turned and looked to see the newspaper partially unwrapped on the ground. Inside was the shattered Star. I spoke without thinking using an impatient, annoyed tone.

"You should pay more attention and be careful!"

How wrong I was. My son was doing a fabulous job but I was too close to see it. His reaction made me ashamed.

During the walk back to the vendor, I had time to think about my behavior. "Dammit how could I be so insensitive?"

"Christopher, I am sorry I got angry and took it out on you."

Like the man I was not, he was understanding and kind. "It's okay dad,"

We bought another one. Each Christmas I look forward to seeing it on the shelf. It serves to remind me to appreciate, be grateful and tolerant.

After arriving in Guayaquil, we travelled to the plane for a short flight to the Islands. The Galapagos is a national park under Federal jurisdiction and controlled by the military. We flew in a small military propeller plane. Young service members in crisp uniforms escorted us to the harbor where our ship rode at anchor.

Once there we walked the dock and boarded a tender boat to ferry us out in the harbor. The dock's long gangway was almost level with the tender because of its shallow draft making it easy to walk on. It brought us out to the moored ship. The cruise ship was an intimate length, more suitable for the area than the mega-ships plying the Caribbean. We pulled up alongside her. In the calmness of the sheltered harbor, the two vessels floated smoothly against one another. The tender was high enough to allow easy access to the ship. It was to be the last simple transfer. After an exhausting day traveling, we got to our cabin. It was an attractive but compact room of rich, polished woods. The ship was small and well appointed, definitely aimed at a refined clientele. We dropped and looked at each other.

"You did it Buddy! You got us here, safe and sound." I exclaimed proudly.

It was quite an accomplishment when broken down to all of the component steps. He handled it beautifully.

"I can't believe we are here." he kept repeating it with each new thing he saw.

"I am so happy we are here too." My grin giving away the excitement I felt.

The eighteen volcanic islands of the Galapagos Archipelago sandwich the equator about 600 miles off the western coast of South America. Few provide a protected harbor. The cruise ship steamed to the offshore reefs circling the islands and dropped anchor. At each stop eager tourists cued up at the hatchway leading to the steep gangplank hugging the side of the ship. We planned to be last at the hatchway to eliminate clogging the line. Christopher donned his bright orange life vest. The sailors helped me. When I stepped through the hatch, my heart sank as I glanced down the narrow, steep steel steps leading down to the water's surface. I clamped onto the handrails and descended each step ever so slowly. By the bottom, my knuckles were white.

Perched just above water level, a rectangular platform provided footing from which passengers stepped off into a wide motor launch. These zodiac style boats were able to bring people all the way up to the edge of the beach. Orange-topped people clung to the ropes lining each side of the boat. They all stared up at my son and me with anticipation. Their expressions were a muddled combination of impatience, support and, I suspect, doubt.

Unlike the first transfer in the sheltered harbor, this one occurred in the open ocean. I stood on the platform above the launch watching it heave several feet as it rode up and down each wave.

"My God," I said under my breath, "How am I ever going to do this without breaking a leg or falling overboard?"

I tensed, surveying the launch, timing the waves and assessing my chances. Christopher stared up at me.

"You can do it, dad. I know you can!"

The sailors closed around me and hands went up to guide me.

"Wait!" I protested.

Wanting to be in control to ensure my safety, I ordered the sailors to assume particular positions on the platform and in the launch. I explained my plan to the sailor in charge who spoke English. He relayed something in Spanish. They all politely listened. Few probably even understood my situation. They smiled and nodded their heads. They were probably laughing at me on the inside. At least they reassured me. The awaiting passengers took it all in wondering, waiting and restless to get going.

My breath quickened with fear. Rationally, I knew I would not drown. An ocean life jacket wrapped around me. Experienced, competent sailors surrounded me. Still, the thought of falling into the ocean or worse yet, landing face first into the launch paralyzed my legs with fear.

"What the hell was I doing out here, thousands of miles from home accompanied only by a 14-year-old boy?" I muttered. "I must have been out of my mind."

I repeated my commands. I timed each passing ocean swell. I gulped and stepped.

"Here goes nothing," I said moving my leg over and went downward.

An unexpected swell passed and the launch dropped three feet. My plans evaporated in the humid tropical air. I was at the mercy of fate.

Arms surged around me and hands gripped my legs, arms and torso. My 6' 2" frame dwarfed the petit Ecuadorian sailors. As if at a rock concert, I found myself body surfing across the sailors, each guiding and moving me through the air towards the launch. Within moments of my step, they placed me safely on the deck amid the raucous shouts of my fellow passengers. I squatted down on the seat, my son smiling broadly at my side.

They transported me through the air and placed me on the launch. The young men in uniform masquerading as sailors in reality were angels.

Similar scenarios repeated several more times as the ship leap frogged from island to island. Each day was a different location. We most often traveled at night to maximize time available to tour. There were no facilities to sleep in the park, meals and lodging were on board the ship.

My son and I stayed with the Aussies and Brits because of the language. Each dinner was a glorious recounting of the day's adventure. Individuals stood describing their experiences and interesting things observed. One evening the unofficial leader of the group stood up and proposed a toast.

"To Chris and his son, who taught us about love, teamwork and survival. You two have shown us the greatest experience of the trip."

My heart filled with pride for my son. How blessed I was to hear this accolade. Those words often return in my memory.

On one island, the group hiked far into the interior over jagged, rough volcanic rock. The distance and terrain made it impossible for me to walk.

I turned to my son, "Sorry, I can't do that, you go."

"No dad, I want to stay here with you," he said.

Christopher and I were 'forced' to hang out on the beautiful, sweeping beach next to a colony of nervous sea lions! As our group disappeared into the fringing forest, a surreal solitude enveloped us. There we sat, strangers in paradise.

The colony returned to their normal activities. The pups and mothers mingled and yakked like parents at a PTA function. They squawked and jabbered as their children scampered about. Off shore a hundred yards, the bulls loudly guarded their families.

Over time, some of the curious pups inched their way closer to us. The moms nervously kept a watchful eye. However, we were the nervous ones. Within thirty yards were several hundred female sea lions each weighing 250 pounds. I grew alarmed as pups approached my child. How would the female react?

A cardinal rule in Galapagos is not to interfere in any way with the natural world. This obviously included touching animals. Christopher looked at me with a mixture of fascination and fear when a pup finally approached him.

"Daddy, what should I do?" as a small pup clambered onto his lap. "I am not supposed to touch the animals. Should I shoo it off?"

"You are a part of the beach. Don't pet it or do anything special. Just sit there and be like a rock, it's okay."

He nestled into his lap and sat there. The little fellow mesmerized us both. His fur was luxurious, the texture of his flippers was smooth and like leather. The eyes were huge and solid black. It had no pupil we could see. I leaned over to snap a photograph.

Satisfied with his investigation, the pup moved on to other adventures. They left us to have our own amazing adventure. We have the photo to prove it.

Other islands held more of Nature's revelations. In a sheltered bay, we snorkeled over tropical reefs. As experienced snorkelers, we were able to dive down a short distance to observe the animals closer. On one dive, we spotted what seemed like missiles darting through the water, a stream of air bubbles trailing behind them. Their appearance was a sudden surprise and they moved so fast it took several moments to identify them. Hypnotized by the swift, graceful path through the water, we watched them cut in and out of the schools of fish all around us.

They were penguins diving to hunt among the fish. The Galapagos Penguin is the only species living north of the equator. The bubbles came from the air trapped in their feathers. Every time they surfaced, air would refill in between the shafts. When they dove again, the pressure compressed the feathers driving out the air as bubbles. As they raced at 20 miles per hour to chase fish, a stream of bubbles followed them. It left a long, moving trail, which slowly rose skyward. It was magical and beautiful to watch.

The saddest thing was being with the last remaining giant tortoise, Lonesome George. The gentle behemoth was a thousand pounds and five feet across. He was the last of his species. The giant tortoise was unable to find mates among the remote and scattered islands. George was alone for years. He finally died a dozen years after we saw him. With his death, the species went extinct. It was a tragic and numbing experience. With other species now protected, their populations have stabilized.

I try to focus on the pleasant, happy memories. Isolation from human contact has produced an absence of fear among many of the animals. I close my eyes and see the comic looking blue-footed booby. Large over-sized bright blue feet set this bird apart. Males strut around like buffoons trying to impress potential mates. It reminded me of my own similar behavior as a parent when I acted like a buffoon. The difference is I should know better.

It was a grand adventure. We welcomed the new year of 2000 sailing on a moonlit Pacific Ocean. All these experiences were possible because of those sailors. The adventures of a lifetime were not in my control. I owe all of it to them.

I had to surrender my will and allow them to do their job unimpeded.

The lesson I learned from this was to trust and give up control. Let go and let God. It is a lesson I am still practicing. For me, it is a tough one to master.

Wind

Around our gardens, my wife and I have several wind chimes. We enjoy sitting outside and hearing them sound. One lazy afternoon their incessant sounding inspired me to write this poem.

Oh, sweet kiss upon my cheek.
So long you have breathed upon us.
Since Zephyrus of Greece, we have held you high.

Yesterday…
Adventurous Vikings beckoned their God, Odin,
"Send the winds," to turn a rising tide.
European explorers aimed their ships for your steady blow to
ply their trade.
Indians on the Plains rejoiced as the majestic Aspen tree
quaked as you brought
the Spring rains and unending buffalo that followed in its
green carpet wake.

Today…
Lobstermen awash in morning mist, await your cleansing
breath.
Imprisoned children seeking park

to escape on the tails of the kite you lift so high.
Even beyond the reach of Earth, manmade intergalactic travelers
Capture your strength in their ingenious solar sails.
Oh, life sustaining wind.

Yet, oh wind, tread lightly with your darkness,
for folk fear your illness:
Shore dwellers stir uneasily when beach grass flattens from an offshore blow.
Young mariners' brides shiver on the widow's walk when a cool,
brisk north wind begins.
Farmers chafe under your unending hot summer whisperings
Hikers search the sky for tale-telling clouds, which blunder your schemes.
Oh, life sustaining wind.

It is no surprise then; we track you close.
Foretold is forewarned!
Beaufort was the first to mark your strength
with his velocity scale.
Vanes are perched high to plot your course.
Chimes placed close will signal your arrival.
We monitor you well,
Oh, life sustaining wind.

Tomorrow....
People, I tell you, hang your own sentinel close:

A melody making mobile. Patiently await its signaling.

Fear not its sounding,
but say,
"Chime for me my sentinel. Cry out, oh Gabriel!"

No ill wind to fear:
It is but an Angel's wing fluttering,
ever attentive, hovering and protecting!
Life giving, life sustaining wind.
Ah, sweet kiss upon my cheek.
Sound incessantly, oh sentinel,
keeping spirits strong.

The lesson in this is not to fear new arrivals. Be open to positive things they may bring. Look at things freshly and don't embrace routine expectations.

Blame The Other Guy

Life often distracts us from questions of eternal importance. Terminal illnesses have a way of re-setting priorities.
For years, I attended Mass on occasion at my parish. Since
my diagnosis, it has become a Sunday routine. My attendance
number in the hundreds. Never once did we experience at
Mass such an inexplicable occurrence.

My wife took a well-deserved weekend getaway, which
set everything in motion. I gave her repeated assurances that I
would be fine when she was gone.

"Honey, I will be okay. Please, don't worry, just go," I
insisted. She needed a break from her constant caregiving
routine.

After much angst, she relented agreeing to leave me with
our young, teenaged son as my caregiver. He and I were on
our own for a father and son weekend. Although this weekend was different from the normal type. I was the one needing
care and supervision. My son became the "in loco parentis."

At that time, my paralysis was not extensive. I had full
use of my legs but not much arm or hand function. I still did
some driving but needed a little help with dressing, eating
and toileting. Beyond that, I was good. Therefore, his responsibilities for my care were not great. The weekend promised
to be a great bonding opportunity.

We "camped in" Friday night. Fast food, kicking back and TV were the evening's fare. Excited by his new role, he rose to expectations. At day's end, he brushed my teeth with care and washed my face. Without losing too much machismo, he undressed me. He tucked me in,

"I love you dad," he told me as he tucked me in bed. He pulled my blanket up, looked down at and grinned.

"Please, tell me a story?" I pleaded referring to our ritual from his early childhood.

He smiled and turned off the light. I drifted off in the quiet darkness recounting with fondness the days when I put him in.

Saturday we spent outdoors working on yard chores. I talked and he worked. It was uneventful, but busy. As we moved from one job to the next, we talked about all sorts of things. I enjoyed hearing his knowledge of science and nature. By the time the day ended, Christopher was exhausted. I think he was glad to see the sun lowering in the sky. We grazed on whatever we found in the fridge. Worn out from the workout I put him through, he wanted to go to bed early. We followed a similar routine as the first evening. We were in bed by ten o'clock. Looking back, he probably wanted his 'parental responsibilities' over.

We are not morning people. We rose late Sunday morning.

"Get up, we are gonna be late for church," I warned him.

He moaned and grunted. "Okay, dad, I heard you," slowly rising from his bed.

Then, the mad rush began. I had to be up, cleaned, shaved and dressed for Mass. Wedged between getting ready and leaving was a quick breakfast. By now, I became work. I

86

think his carefree adolescence seemed a great life when compared to responsibilities of adult caregiving.

"Only one more day, Christopher. Can you hang in there?" I asked.

His answer was, "Hey dad, where are your good pants?"

Of course, we could not find unwrinkled slacks. Getting my limp arms into a dress shirt was much tougher than Saturday's t-shirt. Even my feet were not cooperating as he eased on each snug dress shoe. Racing, we gobbled some toast and beverage, which he prepared in his copious free time. To help make our life easier, my wife filled out a check for the donation basket. She left it in an envelope marked in large letters, "For Church—DO NOT FORGET."

As we scrambled through the door, I barked last minute orders to my harried son.

"Get the keys. Bring my wallet. Make sure you get the envelope," I said in rapid fire.

Demands bombarded the poor kid. I was more a drill sergeant rather than a dad speaking. I heaped my needs and requests on someone else this time. My wife was the usual one to bear the burden made by my needs. This weekend she was free and it was my son's turn.

He ran ahead to open my truck door for me. I lumbered up and over into the seat and he closed the door. He slid across the passenger seat and inserted the ignition key.

For several months, I drove on borrowed time. My fingers were so weak that I could no longer turn the key. I fabricated an oversized key holder giving me better leverage. It allowed me to turn the key again. This solution lasted a short while.

Afterward someone had to start the car for me. Once in a parking lot of a store I couldn't start my truck.

"Uumm, excuse me, can you please help me start my car," I asked a person walking near the truck.

"What do you need?" they replied. My answer left them dumbfounded.

"I need you to turn my key."

The man looked at me in confusion. He was probably thinking, "Is this guy for real?"

"Why?" he asked with suspicion.

I realized how odd my request sounded. "Well, I have trouble with my fingers," not wanting to disclose the full extent of my limitations. "I have Lou Gehrig's disease." I explained. Reassured I was not going to rob him and I was not drunk, he agreed to help.

Christopher leaned over to my side and twisted the key. We were off. Because of my arms, the turns grew hard to maneuver. When we came to the first sharp turn, I asked for his help.

"Slide over Christopher. You can help me with the turns." He enjoyed sitting next to me and "driving."

"This reminds me of my dad when I was a young boy. We used to drive together and he let me hold the wheel. I was thrilled doing it," I shared with Christopher the first time I needed his help.

It is one of the few good memories I have being close to my father. I didn't have a close relationship with him. It is something that I missed. I wanted a different and better one with my son. I wanted to matter in his life. As a result, I tried to be actively involved Dad. ALS abruptly interfered with my plan.

We pulled into the parking lot ten minutes late. Like a tag team, we parked and got out. Anxious about being late, I pushed him to rush.

"Let's go. Let's go,"

I wanted to avoid the embarrassment of the stares late arrivals get.

Nearing the church doors I asked, "You have the envelope, right?"

In a subdued voice he confessed, "I forgot!"

"WHAAAAT?" I wailed. "How could you forget?" I roared in anger, "I told you as we were leaving, don't forget the envelope."

"I'm sorry Daddy," he said. "We were rushing."

I scolded, "You need to think more and be more careful. I am tired of you always forgetting stuff."

His pace slowed and head lowered under my insensitive berating. I huffed away to further show my displeasure. Thoughts of embarrassment consumed me because when the collection basket came to me, I had nothing to put in. Pride made me act selfishly and so harshly.

I waited in the vestibule, staring at him with icy eyes to reinforce my anger. The poor kid. I was so insensitive at the time. We settled in at the end of a back row. Almost no one noticed our arrival. As others communed with God, I remained self-absorbed in false pride. I was foolish and focused on having no envelope for the collection basket. I acted badly in God's House.

It was time I learned a thing or two.

"So, you are worried about being embarrassed, are you? You are angry at your son forgetting the envelope, correct?" I imagined God saying, "Well, let me fix that."

I continued to sit stewing in my silliness. During Mass, the usher came to me tapping me on the shoulder.

"Will you please help us by taking up the collection today?" he asked. Flabbergasted, I turned towards him.

"Umm," stalling to think, "Sorry, I can't. I am disabled."

I could not believe what just happened. No one ever in all the years of attending Mass asked me to be an usher. To reinforce the point God continued the lesson. A second question came from the usher.

"Well, maybe your son would like to do it for you?" the usher suggested.

I shrugged my shoulders more out of disbelief than uncertainty. I looked toward my son whose eyes were now wide and sparkling.

"Sure," he popped. With this, the usher left.

I continued looking at Christopher. His face became serene, no smirk or gloating grin. It was a plain look radiating innocent, forgiving love. If I take the metaphor a bit further, it is the way God smiles at us when we fail to be decent human beings. He loves us unconditionally.

At the appropriate time, Christopher stood and joined the other men at the rear of the church. He got his basket and assignment. He was to collect in my section. The long wicker basket was almost his height. He stretched to his maximum in order to reach into the far end of the pews. I studied him with righteous pride. He progressed down the pews finally reaching mine. I looked at him as he prepared to extend the basket down my aisle.

"God is good," I said in a quiet, humbled voice.

My son slid the basket over towards me. He smiled for an instant as he moved on to the others alongside me.

My empty, false pride burned in my throat. My impatience shamed me, as did my deflection of responsibility. After Mass, I stopped Christopher about where I raved like a lunatic an hour earlier.

"Christopher, I want to apologize for getting mad at you and telling you to be more responsible. It was not your fault we were late and rushing. I should not have been so worried about arriving late or the collection."

I asked God for forgiveness. "Please give me the strength to be a better man."

I also asked my son, "Please forgive me, you are doing a terrific job. I am proud of you."

I thought of a passage from the Bible. "This is my beloved son in whom I am well pleased."

The lesson in this was children have a quick, forgiving, unconditional love, which many adults have lost.

Washed Up: A Tale Retold

I heard a parable inspired by an essay written by Loren Eiseley, which was delivered at an award ceremony for community service. My background in science and my love of the ocean called to me to write a realistic story about taking action against ALS:

Once, a grandfather took his young granddaughter to the seashore for a visit. During the preceding night, a wicked Nor'easter hammered the coast. It piled huge waves on the beach. Atlantic coastal communities know too well the enormous, destructive power these storms can generate.

No sooner had the man eased his car between the lines of the parking lot closest to the beach when the child bolted and raced to the water's edge.

"Grandfather, Grandfather, Come quickly. What are these?" she called out.

Scattered about her feet were the drying carcasses of starfish. The powerful storm wrenched them from the ocean floor. The evening's angry waves hurled them on the beach. The retreating tide marooned them on the dry sand. They baked in the glaring mid-day sun. An irregular swath of dead or dying starfish littered the beach as far as the young girl's eye could see. Filled with disbelief, she questioned her grandfather.

"What happened Grandfather?"

Sensing her distress, he responded with a kind and even, matter of fact tone. "Well, sweetheart," he began, "they were washed up." He detailed how the previous night's strong waves tore up the ocean floor ripping the starfish from the bottom and hurled them onto the beach. He concluded with a last fact about the event.

"It was nature's way," he said.

"But, they're just gonna die?" she echoed. The young girl was unmoved with his explanation and pressed him to know if they *had* to die. She pushed.

She asked repeatedly, "Is there *something* we can do to help them?"

Her wise and sensitive grandfather knelt down with his arm around her and tried to explain with as much tact as possible. He knew that fate had cast its lot and the starfish were doomed. They could do nothing that would make a difference.

Unwilling to accept his fatalistic response, she bent down and picked up one. Turning it over in her palm, she saw the hundreds of tiny tube feet that lined the five arms. Each wriggled as it struggled to right itself in her hand. Holding its life within her fingers, she made an instant decision. Pivoting her body and snapping her arm, she sent the star shooting through the air toward the water. The splash triggered a huge grin. She proceeded continuing to stoop, stand and throw. In a variation of skipping stones, the girl wiled away the afternoon skipping starfish back to the sea, delighting herself as she did.

Off in the distance, a beachcomber approached. From his far-off perspective, all he could see of the pair were the two shapes silhouetted against the horizon. He observed the smaller figure alternating between crouching and standing. As he drew closer, he realized the girl was throwing something in the water. When he reached them, he saw the objects were the dying starfish. He paused, and bid the two a good morning.

"Why are you doing that?" he asked. He was curious why the girl was throwing them.

"Because they'll die if I don't," she shot back, annoyed at the stupidity of the question. The jogger, like the grandfather earlier, tried to explain the situation. He pointed out that stretched all along the beach for miles were untold numbers of starfish. With care, he tried to make her realize she was wasting her time.

"What you are doing will not make any difference."

Undeterred, the girl picked up another starfish and held it in her hand bringing it close to the jogger's face. In silence, they both watched its squirming, wriggling feet slowly twisting. After a moment, the girl flung that starfish out into the water too.

"Think I made a difference to that one, huh?"

We get an opportunity each day. We have the privilege and responsibility of standing amidst some struggling starfish. In everyone, especially an ALS patient, we can see wriggling feet and twisting arms struggling to survive. How we choose to respond to them will make ALL the difference. You may be their last hope. You certainly can make a difference.

Indeed, you must!

Robert Kennedy immortalized the words 'Some see things and ask why. I dream of things and ask why not.'

The lesson I learned from this was conventional wisdom is often an impediment to change. Effort is not wasted if someone or some thing benefits. Don't let negativity discourage you from making a difference.

Somewhere in Time

Elizabeth is my favorite aunt. She is the last of my mother's generation still living. She is the youngest sibling. When my grandmother lived with my family in an upstairs apartment, my aunt was there. I was a toddler. We remained close over the years.

She visited me shortly after Patrick was born in 2007. I just finished the grueling Ride that left me completely exhausted. I did not feel well and stayed in bed for several days. The day before my aunt came, my daughter brought my new grandson over to see me and boost my sagging spirits. The instant I saw the tiny bundle, I felt so much better. He was the best medicine I had. I was lying in bed and Melissa placed him on me.

"Patrick, here's your grandfather," she announced.

All swaddled, he rested in my bosom comfortable and content. I felt wonderful. My spirits indeed lifted. It worked like a magic elixir.

"Hey little fella, how are you?" I asked Patrick. "It's wonderful to see you. Welcome!"

I rallied fast. By morning, I was ready to get up and resume my normal activities.

Elizabeth timed her visit to perfection. I was able to be up and spend time with her. I crowed to her about my happy visit from Patrick.

"He laid on my chest and was so peaceful. He was content and slept," I crowed.

I bragged about his excellent disposition, rambling on like a typical new grandfather. I noticed she was not reacting as I expected. She looked peculiar. It made me stop sooner than I intended. There was an awkward pause while my Aunt silently relived what I described. Finally, Elizabeth broke the silence.

"You never knew your grandfather. He died shortly after you were born," she began.

I listened and nodded in agreement. I acknowledged her with, "I remember hearing stories about him."

My mother spoke about her father often, so I was aware he died from a debilitating lung disease soon after my birth but nothing more. My aunt was only a teenager when it happened.

My words encouraged her, so she continued.

"For his last few years he had great trouble breathing. When you were born, he was bedridden and on an oxygen mask. In many ways, you remind me of him."

"I didn't know that," I replied with surprise. This revelation and its haunting similarities staggered me. I had no idea that happened. My mother died two years before my diagnosis. My grandfather's last days never came up. My aunt added further unbelievable details.

"Your mother was so happy when you were born. As soon as she got out of the hospital, she brought you over to see our father and boost his spirits. He was in bed under a mask struggling to breathe. When she put you on him, you stayed silent on his chest. He lit up and smiled." He died not too long after.

"Wow!" I managed to blurt out, almost speechless.

Now I understood her reaction. The awkwardness returned. We moved on to lighter topics. We talked about family, weather, my work on the charity and ended with our plans for the summer. After a big hug, she left.

I was not sure if I was upset or honored being a special branch in this tree of life. When she left, my wife tried to put everything in perspective for me. The bewilderment remained.

Six decades separated these events. The similarities were uncanny. Two terminally ill grandfathers, each having lung problems that required mechanical breathing support requiring masks. Both were bedridden. Our daughters sought to cheer us with their recently delivered baby. Unable to sit, the babies nestled on our chests.

The last and most striking to me involved our names. My daughter liked the name Patrick. She named her son Patrick Christopher (Christopher was in honor of me). My mother named me Christopher in honor of her father. As my aunt told the story, she revealed my grandfather's full name - Christopher Patrick. My grandson's name was a mirror image, Patrick Christopher.

Loving daughters link all three of us—generations of Christophers.

It must have been a bittersweet memory for my aging aunt. I am sure she was as moved as I was. We never referred to the experience again.

The conversation left me unsettled. I did not understand my feelings. I wrestled with whether it meant something. I came to terms by accepting not everything has an explanation.

The Serenity Prayer helped me find peace. I rewrote it for the circumstance.

> *God grant me the serenity*
> *to accept the things I cannot understand,*
> *the courage to cope with the things I can*
> *and wisdom to know the difference.*

Unlike my unfortunate grandfather, I have lived many happy years with my grandson. We shared countless joys together. When I pass, I hope Patrick recalls me with love and the priceless gift we had-time. He and I were quite lucky.

The lesson I learned from this was there is a surreal, mystical connection among families, which spans generations. It defies understanding. It merely requires acceptance.

Angels Among Us

So much of my life depends upon help from people of all walks of life. How fortunate I am to have people in my life who care. I wrote this poem to recognize my caregivers and the myriad of others who care.

Among all of *the world* there is so much need, yet
Nobody today *seems* to have the time or desire to help.
Going full steam, *so* much is left behind racing through life.
Each is very *self-absorbed*; they ignore the cries for help
Luckily, *a few* slow down to grab an outstretched hand.
Some, *like you, still care* about others.

The lesson in this was people who help others are special and possess great empathy. They make a difference in our lives. The world is a better place due to those who take the time to care.

Men, Medicine and Miracles

My heart broke for many reasons following my diagnosis with ALS. As much as I thought about what I would lose to this paralyzing ailment, I also thought about what I would never have. The life expectancy of a typical ALS patient is so short. I assumed my life would be significantly shortened. High school graduations, weddings and grandchildren were things I would never know. I would die in the prime of my life. But there is a saying, "as man plans, God decides."

Beyond all realistic hope, I was there to see my daughter graduate college. I attended my son's high school and college graduation. To my delight, I walked Melissa down the last ten feet of the aisle at her wedding.

In time, I held my baby grandson nestled all secure between my knees as I sat in my wheelchair. I rolled around showing him off through the neighborhood on my morning "walk". The warm summer sun shined on us and the world was indeed good. I excitedly looked forward to winter and our first Christmas together.

While everyone else was celebrating the joys of the holiday season, my grandson Patrick was collapsing further into the clenches of what we thought to be a worsening respiratory infection. Our daughter, Melissa, and my wife played phone tag, relaying the latest temperature reading or activity level.

His food intake, which had always been a problem, was down to a sparse two or three ounce feeding. He did not look, nor act, as a typical seven-month old baby boy. In medical terms, he wasn't thriving. My daughter shuttled him back and forth to the pediatrician.

By New Years, he all but stopped eating and his temperature remained high at 103. For most of New Year's Day, he lay quiet, content in someone's arms. For all the noise and commotion around him, his stillness was troubling.

The fever continued to inch ever upward. On January 2, it became quite high and nothing seemed to break it. I asked a nurse friend, Mary Pat, to stop by their house and take a look at him. After seeing his lethargic condition, the two discussed options. He began projectile vomiting and pushed the pair into action. Mary Pat soothed Patrick as Melissa threw a few things together and they bolted for the emergency room of a community hospital, St. Charles. Expecting news about a bad respiratory infection or maybe pneumonia, they were unprepared for the ordeal to come.

After a quick assessment, the doctors at St. Charles suggested we send Patrick to Stony Brook University Hospital, a regional medical center of excellence, because it was a more appropriate treatment center for infants. They explained Patrick had a high white blood cell count.

"Your son's blood count is over 70,000," the staff told Melissa.

My daughter's blank stare in response to the count (which is a life threatening level) revealed her failure to grasp the dimension of the developing crisis facing Patrick.

"Okay, now what?" she asked.

"Stony Brook University Hospital would be the best place, 'just in case' anything developed." They described how Stony Brook was better for young children.

"They have all the equipment. They are a better facility for your son." The ER staff ordered an ambulance transfer STAT. After hearing the news, my son-in-law, Craig, raced to Stony Brook. Stunned by the developments, we didn't know a bomb was about to detonate.

St. Charles sent over his records. Upon arrival at the second ER, a prearranged medical team appeared from nowhere and swarmed over Patrick like pack of wolves defending a pup. They whisked him straight to pediatric intensive care. Craig and Melissa stared in disbelief as an ocean of green scrubs swallowed their baby.

By that time, it was near midnight when my wife arrived to lend moral support. Mary Pat arrived, her nursing background proving a valuable ally. She bridged the informational divide between medicine and patient. I had to stay at home. The situation worsened. The five at the hospital realized by the intensity and range of activity that something other than a bad respiratory infection was going on.

Out of the din, one ER doctor emerged. "Patrick's records and x-rays were sent via a computer to the home of their pediatric surgeon," he announced. "He read them and was coming to the hospital right away." The ER doctor continued, "The surgeon suspected Patrick needed emergency surgery."

"Why," Craig asked, "we thought he had a respiratory infection."

"We think your son has a diseased colon that has become severe. It has to be removed." When Dr. Scriven arrived, he confirmed his diagnosis.

"We need to take it out right away," he said in a serious, clear voice.

"But it is 1 AM!" Melissa said in protest.

"The infection has spread throughout his body. We need to remove it now. Your son is a very sick baby," he said.

We hurtled from expecting cough syrup to surgery at warp speed. It turned out Patrick had an easily detectable but undiagnosed birth defect called Hirschsprungs disease. During fetal development, the growing nerve cells did not develop as they should. They did not reach the far end of the colon. Thus, without nerve endings the colon muscles can't rhythmically contract to move the stool along.

Without this contraction, his bowel movements became irregular and stool accumulated in the colon causing it to distend. If discovered early, it is treatable without serious complications. In Patrick's case, it went unrecognized and did extensive damage to his large intestine.

His chronic constipation was due to a functional obstruction caused by the birth defect. Over time, his colon suffered permanent damage. His colon had distended so much that the tissue began to die. That damage became infected bringing him to the brink of death.

The blood picked up the bacteria and spread it throughout his body. Patrick was under a massive, body-wide infectious assault. We were fortunate St Charles sent him to University hospital. Our baby was in an epic battle for his life. There was no better place to make his stand and fight to live. It came to involve the best most, dedicated medical personnel in the area.

Dr. Scriven came out after a couple of hours. Melissa and Craig ran over to talk.

"The surgery went well under the circumstances. I took out half his colon. He is resting."

"How is he?" she asked.

"Well, he is stable at the moment. His incision was not closed."

"Why is he not closed?" she said in bewilderment.

"I want to see how he does. We need to control the infection. The piece of colon I left in looks salvageable but we have to see."

"So, where is he now?" not understanding the entire procedure going on.

"He is still in the OR. I draped the incision in sterile wrapping. We put him on a bunch of powerful antibiotics to stop the infection."

"What happens next?" she asked, terrified to hear the answer.

"If we can stop the infection, we connect everything back and close him up." He explained to the group that Patrick had to improve before they close him. "His colon was in bad shape. I didn't want to take everything at once because of the consequences."

"What do you mean by consequences?" Melissa pressed.

"If I took it all I would condemn him to a life using an ostomy bag. He has his whole life ahead. I didn't want to do that unless it's the last resort."

Melissa cried as she took it all in. Craig asked the next step.

"What will you do now?"

"We wait to see how the drugs work."

Even though it was nearly morning, the surgeons remained close to monitor their tiny patient. As the hours dragged by, instead of showing improvement, his condition worsened. The drugs were unable to control the system-wide infection gripping his body. The team debated how best to treat Patrick. As his clinical signs deteriorated, there was no other choice.

Dr. Scriven came out six hours after his initial surgery and delivered the bad news.

"The drugs are not working. I have to go back and remove all of it to save him."

They rushed him back to remove his entire large intestine and thus any source of further infection. Then Dr. Scriven disagreed with his partner. He refused to give up on saving a tiny bit of tissue. He worked feverishly to clean and preserve a small stump above his rectum.

He came out to report to the family, "I did 'everything' that medical science could do."

The baby's kidneys were shutting down, the respiration shallow and rapid. It taxed his heart, sending it racing. His dehydration combined with the infection caused his veins to collapse. The only working IV the nurses could use went into his tiny, bald head. Through it poured a cocktail of potent antibiotics that also threatened him. He was on life support and critically ill. Modern medicine had done its best. They were hopeful the drugs would be able to control the infection.

The big question: would the drugs have enough time to be effective.

"It is up to Patrick to fight," he concluded.

He must hang on long enough to give the medication time to work. We sent desperate calls for prayer by person, phone, and computer. Father Frank Pizzarelli, our family priest who married Craig and Melissa was on a trip to the Holy Land.

"I will pray at the Wailing Wall in Jerusalem for Patrick," he promised in an email.

My Pacific Islander caregiver called home to have her father a minister pray with his Fiji congregation. My computer network of ALS friends and patients throughout the country were monitoring and praying. People stretching half way around the globe joined the struggle to help keep baby Patrick alive through their prayers. We held our breath, prayed and waited.

A true stubborn Taurus, Patrick clung to his medical lifelines. As each hour passed, our hopes grew. Within twenty-four hours, the tide began to turn. By forty-eight hours, his color improved; his kidneys started producing. By seventy - two hours, his white blood count began a significant decrease. Within days, the fever broke and he was breathing on his own. When we spoke with the doctor on the third morning, he used a new term.

For the first since he took the case, Dr. Scriven said, "When Patrick gets better!" Up to then, in countless conferences he always said with caution, "If Patrick pulls through."

From that moment on, we knew Patrick would live.

The next four months remained a nightmarish blend of infection and re-hospitalization and endless adjustments to a shifting medical situation. His infection was a virulent, drug resistant, C-Dif. Scriven consulted everyone in his struggle to save his little patient. The head of Infectious Diseases guided the effort to arrest the resilient infection. During January and half of February, most nights were spent in the hospital. His mom or dad juggled and alternated overnight shifts while the grandparents pulled some of the day duties.

Sometimes, I got lucky and could go. I loved being with him but it was not easy to see. Attending the needs of a critically sick infant awash with tubes, catheters and monitors, is a task not easily done.

After an eternity, Patrick went home with a plastic bag attached to the side of his belly that held his stool. Emptying his ostomy bag replaced changing diapers. He wormed and fidgeted across the mattress as his parents struggled to change the bag half his size glued securely to his side. For a long time, he had a central port line deeply embedded into his chest, which emptied directly into a large blood vessel near his heart. The aorta artery provided enough blood flow needed to dilute the toxic brew of the unending round-the-clock numerous IV treatments he received.

It was a difficult time for the family. There were more surgeries and midnight ER visits. The surgeon wound up coming to the house, like the country doctors used to do a generation ago. It spared Patrick and my daughter from the exhausting and dangerous trips to the hospital.

Melissa learned to irrigate the stoma, the site where his intestine stuck out of his belly. She perfected probing through it into his small intestine. She had to dislodge blockages that formed. The Scali dining room looked like a mobile crash unit similar to what the military used in Iraq or Afghanistan. They struggled to stay one-step ahead of a drug resistant bacterium. All the while, our friends and family prayed.

By the end of April, he was finally infection free. In May, Dr. Scriven began some reconstructive surgery on his one-year-old patient. On July 29, he had what we hope will be Patrick's last procedure. Using the small rectal stump he fought so hard to save, he created a small pouch. Pulling the small intestine, he attached it to the stump forming a continuous pathway. Four days later, we received a phone call from Melissa.

"Patrick pooped!" she screamed into the phone.

In a normal home, such an occurrence is not cause for celebration but with him, it was six months in the making. Who would guess the joy a dirty diaper would bring! The strong acids made the liquid stool quite caustic, burning Patrick's behind, making diaper changes painful. For a time, his bum oozed like a hot pizza pie.

"His body will adjust and adapt. In time his stool will thicken some," she said adding, "his skin will toughen and not be as tender."

I asked, "Will he have any control?"

She said, "According to the doctor, he will learn to control himself to a large degree."

That was better than any of us dare dream a few months ago. Barely four weeks after reconstruction, Patrick was playing, walking, babbling, eating and most importantly, pooping quite like any toddler. Looking at his smile, one would never know. He grew and thrived.

Now on some Saturday mornings, I rise extra early and rush my caregiver to get me ready to go out. We drive to a local ice rink to watch ice hockey. I scan the ice for the player with number three on his jersey. I can no longer shout Patrick's name, I do scream on the inside like the proud grandpa I am as he glides gracefully down the ice. He does a bit of fancy stick handling when sees his Poppy on the other side of the Plexiglas. I flash a big smile back.

I share our story about life saving and restoration as something to think about. It was a case that should have gone the other way. In fact, at first when things looked the grimmest, Craig and Melissa turned to the surgeon for solace. They sought some reassurance. They wanted the doctor to give a prediction of things to come.

"Tell us the truth. What are his chances?"

"I don't know. No patient I treated lived this long."

The surgeon didn't have an answer because, in his experience with a case this advanced, no other patient survived. When it was all over, he said, "Patrick was in a league of his own."

Survive he did. His future will present many challenges, but he is alive to face them. For those close to Patrick who know the entire story, it is a miracle.

Through an incredible series of circumstance, he wound up in the care of an extraordinary medical facility. Marvelous doctors, nurses and medical staff treated him. He had the benefit of the latest technologies. Yet with it all, his survival was still questionable.

In the twilight between living and dying exists a world we know little about. Why was Baby Patrick able to cling to life during the hours following his second surgery with failing organs and on life support? Medical workers have a dark expression referring to patients critically ill and not expected to live. They are 'circling the drain.'

How did he manage to circle the drain long enough and not be sucked down? Why didn't the massive infection already squeezing the life out of him not continue its march to his death? What was it that sustained his life when his body could not?

The off-the-cuff answer? Well, he was one lucky little boy.

When Baby Patrick entered twilight, he was escorted through the shadows. Like everyone, he headed towards the bright light at the end of the tunnel. Then he turned around. He took the path back toward life. Luck had little to do with it. Our family knows why. We have no doubts.

Prayer illuminated the path he followed through the darkness. Prayers lit his way back like an airport's bright runway beacons showing a plane the way to safety on a foggy night.

His sojourn into the night turned out to be a loop rather than straight path, thank God.

If Baby Patrick could have thanked everyone himself, he would. Since he was only fifteen months old, I said it for him.

"Thank you, Dr. Scriven. Thank you to the pediatric surgery team, and the angels who staff PICU at Stony Brook University Hospital."

To those who helped him cling to life and kept the airport lights on through their prayer. "Thank you to the army of people who prayed."

It reinforces what I said as I began, "Man plans, but God decides."

The lesson I learned from this was medicine is indeed an art. Doctors do their best and that is all they can do. The rest is out of their hands. Into whose hands does it fall? Sometimes there are no explanations for why things occur. Prayer is as valid as any other.

Dedicated to the men and women who toil each day
to lessen suffering and bring hope to the sick.
In particular, this salutes those who tend to the tiniest
in Pediatric ICUs across the nation.

The Voice

My disease is uncommon. None of my family, friends or I knew anyone with it. Early in its course, I felt awash without a sense of community. Experience taught me the importance of feeling connected, not isolated and alone. A friend received a diagnosis with a return of her breast cancer after some years. I wrote this tale to boost her spirits. Perhaps it would give her a sense of support. I hoped the story would strengthen her resolve to battle once again.

Once upon a time, a woman strolled in the park enjoying a beautiful sunny day. From nowhere, a tap pressed her shoulder. Startled, she spun around to investigate but no one was there. Perplexed, she paused. Could it have been her imagination?

With similar mystery, the Voice boomed. It directed her to the end of the park. The resonating, transfixing voice ushered her forward. She arrived amidst a gathering to discover a race was to start. The Voice spoke again and instructed her to run. This is crazy she thought.

"I am not going to run," she protested under her breath. "First, I am not a good runner and secondly, I am just out for a stroll. I am not even dressed for a run."

She wondered if she was nuts. However, The Voice was quite real and commanding to her. Somehow, she felt compelled to comply. Against her will, she yielded and began to run.

Numerous runners jostled and jammed the narrow course, making progress difficult. She focused on the path ahead, deciding to do what was necessary to complete the race. To her surprise, she encountered bystanders who cheered her. As the miles dragged on, fatigue settled in. Each time her energy dropped or spirit sagged, The Voice spoke encouragement. She listened and responded with renewed effort. Midway, she realized the course was perfect in design. A gentle gliding slope followed each difficult hill. It enabled her to coast for short sections. The woman manufactured enough resolve to persevere.

After a long, arduous journey, the finish line loomed ahead. Ecstatic and relieved, her unwanted ordeal was about to end. However, things are not always, as they appear. At the conclusion of the foot race, The Voice called out to her still again.

"You are not finished. There is more for you to do."

"I am finished with you, leave me alone!" shouted the bewildered woman, "I am done. I will not do anything else, do you hear me?"

Ignoring her pleas and denials, the Voice commanded she continue. "You must proceed to the lake. Now you have to swim," The Voice instructed.

She protested again, "But, I am not interested in swimming,"

First, she was not a swimmer and secondly, she was exhausted from the run. However, as before, The Voice was quite demanding and she was obliged to comply. With the will of a hungry lion, the woman dove into the lake. When she hit the water, the clothes weighed her down. It was a struggle to keep her head above water.

Her ordeal began anew. A steady wind swept the surface of the lake, challenging her progress. Every time she rotated her head on each stroke, wavelets slapped her face. They insulted her body as the unwanted race had violated her will. Yet, she plodded onward. When she held her head high clearing the water's surface, she could see people wave from the shore. With methodic, rhythmic strokes, she crossed the lake toward a sandy spit jutting from the shoreline. It formed a small cove.

Along the finger of sand reeds lined the shallow water of the cove. The stand of cattails swayed in the wind, as if waving her a welcome. As she skirted the tall, green sentinels guarding the shore, a chorus of croaking frogs greeted her. Like a police officer on escort duty, one huge bullfrog hopped off a nearby lily pad and moved alongside the spent swimmer. Delighted by her new companion, she found the strength to match the frog stroke for stroke. They covered the remaining few yards together. The frog stayed in the lake, sitting at the water's edge.

The swimmer emerged from the water and inched up the sloping sand, dropping to her knees. She collapsed on the grass of the far shore. The ground cushioned her as she sprawled, her body wracked with pain and drained from exhaustion. Unable to lift her head, she sheltered it in her arms. She laid motionless.

She listened for the Voice. There were no sounds. The Voice was silent. The race was indeed over. She made it.

Realizing her unwanted ordeals were completed, she flushed with serenity. At that moment, the bullfrog croaked an approval from the water's edge.

Are you not also in an unwanted race for your life? Remember, things are not as they seem. You have to compete in a biathlon for life. You did not have one but two events to finish. In ways, this second challenge will be more difficult to complete. However, you are now a seasoned competitor. You have gained inner strength, which will steel you. Move with confidence and courage. Go forward, friend.

A glorious love and appreciation of life replace the things taken away. Look and you will see your path paved by insights you have developed. You will successfully finish this course as well. Have no doubt.

Everyone is racing somewhere. Many have no idea where they are going or why. As mice on an exercise wheel, they race in circles. Unlike them, you are running for a purpose. You can do it. You can do it.

Understand, the Voice will always demand someone run the race. On occasion, it is a biathlon. There are no volunteers in this race. Use your positive energy to move along to the finish line. Stay focused on what is in front. Listen to the cheers of bystanders along the way. They want to see you win! Aim for the frog, she is waiting to help you.

After giving the story to my friend, she called me. She loved the story. It did lift her spirits. She wondered why I chose a frog for the metaphor.

"Was there any particular reason you chose a frog for the story?" she asked.

"No, I just like frogs," I told her.

Then she asked me, "Do you know what FROG represents?"

"I didn't know it represented anything," I answered with curiosity.

To my utter disbelief, she informed me, "It stands for Forever Rely On God!

Why was I so surprised? Whenever I pass a pond or hear a frog croak, I smile.

The lesson I learned from this was life-altering challenges will confront everyone. We can't select the one we want but we can decide how we respond. You don't take on the challenge alone. People are encouraging you to keep fighting. A higher power is behind you.

Transcending

I heard that fear is nothing more than the absence of hope. I gave this some thought and came up with this poem. It is about moving from fear to hope.

Few notice **I**ts presence: masked in stealt**H**,
Embedded throughout, it ri**n**gs like a lass**O**.
Attack and work **t**o loosen its choking gri**P**.
Rely on faith and there y**o**u will find peac**E**.

The lesson I learned from this was fear is pervasive. It chokes victims, paralyzing them. Turn to faith and fight to turn fear into hope, which brings peace.

Blind Date

In the beginning, darkness covered the world until God created light. In time, a great storm rose up and laid waste to all the island. The seas rose to a mighty height and evil, wicked winds blew. The land blackened once more. Great lament spread through the darkness. Hurricane Sandy had come to wrought her destruction. She laid waste to the land and departed.

The New York Governor Cuomo cameth and said, "Let there be light."

And behold, a powerful surge pulsed once more through the island. Then he proclaimed, "It was good."

Following this great wonder, the Governor rested and did nothing.

Only the chosen were blessed on that first day, for many still languished in the dark. On the seventh day cameth back the lights and the sacred screen shown through the empire of New York. We hadith power and we leapt with joy, exalting our deliverance. For indeed, LIPA (Long Island Power Authority) liveth, and salvation was at hand. Peace began to reign everywhere in the land of milk and honey.

"Glory be to God and his trusted servant, Cuomo," shouted the satisfied throngs.

Lo, discourse still remained in the lines of those gathered to worship idols at the gas temples. There greed, anger and gnashing of teeth prevailed. Cuomo could perform signs and wonders, but for Pete's sake, he wasn't God. Restoring gasoline, the mana of automobiles would take a higher power. Such a miracle was beyond pay grade of a public servant.

The Pendergast family rejoined the world after an adventurous seven-day stint living in the post-modern era: sans electric. During our time without power, we fired up the woodstove for warmth.

"Let's use our old camping gear." I suggested. I saved some equipment from our camping days eons ago.

"Who knows if those relics still work," Christine responded.

We dragged a rusted, dusty propane camping stove caked with old food left overs and a dented lantern.

"I don't remember how they work." She never was big on roughing it.

"I have small cylinders of propane in the garage," I said. "Get 'em, they screw in. It's easy," I assured her.

"Wow, they still work!" she said.

I was not sure if she was relieved or disappointed at the prospect of reliving our camping glory days. Most importantly, we lined up a formidable array of batteries to run my ventilator non-stop. We had heat, light and a stove, albeit crude. I could breathe for the time being.

"What more could we ask for?" I said half-serious.

We settled in, bundled up, kept one eye on the battery indicator, the other on the thermometer. We said our prayers by candlelight of necessity.

Near dusk on the day the hurricane struck, just before its full fury, our son in law, Rich, Melissa, Patrick and I had ventured down our street to the bluffs overlooking the Long Island Sound. We wanted to see and feel nature at her most powerful. The wind roared like an angry lion as it torn the sky above us. The treetops appeared like puppets dancing out of control. They bent and twisted in the wind.

The gale beat the water on the Sound to a meringue froth. An army of marching waves plowed into the shore. The ravenous water bit into the sand at the base of the cliff, devouring huge chunks with each bite. The storm consumed the cliff. Large sections of the top toppled over, threatening the homes on the cliff. It was as murderous as it was majestic. We lost our power soon after we returned.

The day after Sandy hit, Rich, a doctor, loaned us a brand new generator. He bought it right before the storm because of concern for my well-being. I guess once a doctor, always a doctor! With the help of our neighbor, Bill Papaleo, we started the generator, running it on and off for power to supply a radio, electric blanket to warm me, keep our refrigerator cold and recharge the crucial ventilator. We put the camping gear back in the garage.

When the temperature nose-dived several days after the hurricane, my brother-in-law came over to show my son how to wire our furnace to the generator. The temporary hook up would get us through the crisis because it gave us the furnace, hot water and heat. We endured the third world reality of rationed power getting only several hours each day because gas to run the generator was impossible to get. Our life revolved around the noisy but welcomed sound of a running generator.

Our salvation was my daughter, Melissa, who never lost power in her home. By luck, she lived nearby and had us over each evening to warm up, charge batteries and have a good meal. After dinner, we played board games. It was fun in a rustic sort of way for a while. However, I was most comfortable at home where I had everything I needed set up. So, each evening we headed back across the divide into the land the Governor and LIPA forgot.

The most memorable image I will keep was the seagulls we saw on our adventure to experience the hurricane. They were also out flying. Perhaps they looked at us with similar surprise. I mused, what brought us both out on such a fierce occasion? I recall their bizarre flight. I tilted my head to see them silhouetted above against the racing clouds. Motionless, wings outstretched, they rode on the winds with ease. They did not fly forward as normal, they glided by *sideways*.

Spellbound, I watched them sliding down the coastline of the bluff. Gull after gull queued up in some unintelligible order, passing overhead following the ferocious flow of the wind. I thought of the gull in my poem. We posed and snapped a photo of us standing at the edge of the cliff, forever anchoring the scene in our mind of the perfect storm.

Thankfully, our loss from Sandy was limited to a couple of black cherry trees. They held our hammock and Patrick's tire swing. We also lost a few sections of the fence they took out. Deadly winds rendered the backyard like a war zone with debris strewn everywhere. Two huge bomb craters marked where the roots once held the trees fast. In the springtime, a new flowerbed would hide the scars and the blooms came to brighten spirits, soothing frightening memories. I have a load of stories, but none as compelling or sad as all those folks who have lost everything, including loved ones. My thoughts and prayers go out to them.

Neil Keating, another Long Island PALS, person with ALS, faced a more threatening situation. He had a tracheotomy and spent much of his time in bed. His aging parents provided most of his care. Worried about their son's safety, they searched for options. To be cautious, the family decided to move him to a hospice center, which was equipped to handle emergencies. After getting Neil, a Suffolk County police officer, settled in and comfortable, they entrusted him to the nursing staff. They left for an uncertain fate in their own vulnerable south shore home near the ocean.

As the storm raged outside, Neil developed difficulties. Tragically, Neil died on the first night, October 11, 2012. His name never appeared on the official storm casualties list. Yet he lost his life because of Hurricane Sandy. Amid their heartache, they thought to share his specialized equipment. With selfless love, his parents distributed Neil's devices to area PALS. I sadly accepted his eye-controlled computer. With it, I began my journey with assistive technology. I used it for several years and presented school assembly programs to thousands of students with his help. Using a second-generation eye gaze machine, I wrote a large part of this book. In a way, Neil is still speaking.

We all attempted to return to our "normal" lives. Thousands lost homes, automobiles and other properties. Years later, some are still dealing with storm aftermath issues.

Their lives will never be regular again. Let us keep those people in mind and prayer.

My date with Sandy was one of my most memorable dates. It reinforced me to remember-hold dear all that is truly important. They are our real, irreplaceable treasures.

The lesson I learned from this was to separate comfort and possessions from the important things in life. I tend to become lost in things but most of them are replaceable. Treasure what are irreplaceable-family and friends.

Art Imitating Life: The Theory of Everything

I have travelled the same road as Stephen Hawking, facing similar issues and challenges brought into our lives by ALS. There were striking similarities. He and I were both long time patients, diagnosed earlier than the average age (21 and 44 respectively). We have lived with the disease well beyond the normal survival time of 2-3 years, although his 51 years dwarfed my 27 years. We were educators. We loved science. Finally, we both actively promoted ALS awareness.

It is understandable why I had a twinge of trepidation when I attended the movie in 2014, The Theory of Everything, an Academy Award and Golden Globe winner. How would I react to a Hollywood conjured representation of a nightmare that I lived each day? How would I feel seeing a personal hero portrayed by some actor trying to interpret our grim realities of living in a body ravished by paralysis juxtaposed with a vivid, robust intellect and a *joie de vivre*?

The movie did not disappoint. Eddie Redmayne was almost picture perfect in his overall accurate portrayal of Hawking. His Academy Award for Best Actor was well deserved. He captured minute details such as the contractures in Hawking's hands due to prolonged muscle spasticity caused by ALS. Redmayne re-created Hawking's iconic body slant, head tilt and smile quite well. His delivery of lines and the contortions made him appear to be a patient, not an actor playing a patient. I marveled at how well Redmayne was able to depict the physical manifestations of the disease.

One of the personally poignant moments was watching him trip and fall while walking on the campus lawn early into my illness. I also experienced those unsettling falling episodes. I fell on my own school campus breaking my leg. Most of the kids and staff were gone. Foolishly, I traipsed through an inviting pile of autumn leaves on the way to the office after school.

I loved the rustling, crunching leaves as I plowed through. They fluffed effortlessly as my legs pushed them up like a snowplow. I stumbled over something hidden by the leaves. I went right down like Redmayne. The leaves engulfed me swallowing me whole. I became invisible to the world. It was as if a black hole sucked me down. I laid in pain calling for help. Luckily, a teacher friend, Brian Ohst, happened to hear my cries and came over to investigate. He neared the leaf pile.

"Chris?" he called recognizing my voice wondering where I was hiding.

"Brian, I am in here!" I cried out in desperation. "Help me."

He bent over and peered into the leaves. To his shock, he discovered me under the leaves rolling in pain

"Oh my God! What happened?"

"I was walking to the office and cut across the lawn and through the leaves. I hit something and it knocked me off balance. I went straight down on top of my leg," I told him.

He pushed aside the leaves and saw the legs bent like pretzels under me. He rolled me and I moaned in pain. We tried standing, but it hurt too much.

"You need to see a doctor," he pronounced.

"Let me lie here awhile," I asked. I didn't want to go to the hospital.

"Go and have it checked out," he insisted. Against my wishes, he dialed 911 and saved me from an unknown fate.

This instability was the final straw that compelled me to see a neurologist. Watching it larger than life on the screen happening to someone else brought my bittersweet flashback. So too was the scene in which he was diagnosed.

Redmayne tried to illustrate the challenges of walking with ALS. The advancing paralysis in Hawking's legs depicted in the film by him walking pigeon toed was one of the few inaccurate scenes I noticed. Patients are unable to walk due to muscle weakness and foot drop. These conditions are nearly impossible for an able-bodied person to mimic in a realistic manner. The actor attempted to create a visual to convey the idea. In real ALS life, walking is much more hesitant, imbalanced and limb dragging. It was a good, though inaccurate, try.

I resonated with the frustration and anger shown in the scene where Hawking was encouraged to use an augmentative communication device. An alphabet board is a frustrating and tedious way to express one's thoughts. The audience has no idea the isolation and terror that scene illustrated. I am now losing my ability to speak and only a few people are able to decipher my words. Thus, watching Redmayne's rejection of the overtures to communicate stung. How will I be able to handle that final day of not speaking when it comes?

Like Hawking, I am independent to a fault and enjoyed the movie's focus on continuing to live despite overwhelming challenges. He raised a family, pursued a career, remain productive and fell in and out of love (the resemblance ended with the latter as I am still in love and married to my childhood sweetheart of 50 years). The audience got a guidebook on living life to its fullest. Hawking is a model for all of us. He demonstrated the limit is beyond the sky! There is no excuse for saying I can't. There is simply no giving up.

My final thoughts concern something underscoring the entire movie. He achieved marvelous things in his life. But, those accomplishments were possible only because he accepted assistance...

One cannot live long with ALS unless willing to embrace help. *Everyone* is universally interdependent. We survive with the help of one another. Paralyzed patients require steadier help. Stephen's wife, Jane, well played by Felicity Jones, was emblematic of caregiver spouses everywhere. They try keeping their loved ones well cared for, focused on the future and enjoying life. During the movie, they carried me to the toilet, fed, dressed and transported me right along with Redmayne. Without my caregivers, I would not be writing this. I am alive, productive and happy because of them. Topping the list of wonderful caregivers I have, is Christine.

I was heartbroken when Stephen and his wife divorced. Successful, long-term marriages are rare today. The Hawkings, under enormous pressure of coping with ALS and public scrutiny, proved no different from many other couples. They divorced. I felt sad as I observed Jane and Stephen grow distant, due in part to the strain of care he required. I watched, understanding the phenomenal stress on Jane. I saw the relationships each developed with others as their own ebbed cold. I wished it wasn't so. I try very hard to ensure my wife maintains a life outside my care. I want to be her partner, not her burden.

With *The Theory of Everything*, moviegoers got a decent, accurate glimpse into the lives of ALS patients. They also got a story about a remarkable man who taught the world about black holes in the limitless universe.

It illustrated that there is a limitless power we all have within regardless of physical limitations.

Is this a case of art imitating life or life imitating art? Go watch the movie and judge for yourself.

One of the many lessons in this was the pivotal role caregivers play in assisting people to maximize their potential. In many cases, it is the spouse leading the way to a productive and happy life for the mate. Unfortunately, it often comes at their own emotional and physical expense.

A Western Tale

When I was a kid back in the late '50s, I grew up watching Westerns. John Wayne's picture appeared everywhere. *Gunsmoke* was the number one TV show. Every show seemed to be about outlaws wearing big black hats robbing a stagecoach or bloodthirsty Native Americans attacking innocent pioneers. In either case, the ending was similar. The sheriff or the Cavalry, both wearing white hats, rode in at the last minute to save the day.

How many times did I watch a wagon train close in a defensive circle to fight off an attack? Usually, besieged pioneers ran out of bullets, their wagons set aflame and the horses shot. In typical Hollywood fashion, the settlers were down for the final count. In perfect timing, off in the distance was heard a faint but growing sound of a bugle. From out of nowhere, the United States Cavalry charged in to the rescue with guns blazing and flags flapping. Within minutes, all was well. In the innocent mind of a child, a wrong righted, good overcame evil and the world was just.

I suppose my family and I may appear as those encircled pioneers, facing an overwhelming, powerful and hostile foe. We fought with every ounce of our strength, exhausted our supplies and resources. Still, the enemy continues the attack. The hopeless situation lingered until we too were down for the last count. When surrender, followed by death, are the only options, what else is there to do but fight on?

"Wait! What is that I hear in the distance?" I question. I strain to hear better. "No, it can't be…this is the real world." I remind myself.

"Honey, do you hear that?" I asked my wife.

"I do, what is it?"

The sound grows louder becoming unmistakable.

"There's a bugle blowing!" she shouts in disbelief. "Is there a Cavalry a coming to our rescue?"

In our real world, we added my new bedroom on the house. For three years, I struggled with the stairs to my old bedroom on the second floor using my weakening legs. The trip was getting more difficult. I reached the point of danger. In Hawking's book, *A Brief History of Time*, it describes him going up the stairs.

A guest was visiting his wife, Jane, and they chatted in the living room. The guest noticed behind Jane, Stephen was crawling up the stairs.

Unable to believe her eyes she asks, "Jane, why is Stephen crawling?"

"Because he can," she said curtly.

I was not far behind Stephen. On the morning news for September 9, 1999, I heard on the news that Catfish Hunter, another Yankee player with ALS, fell down his staircase and died from injuries.

I said to my wife, "That is not going to happen to me if I can help it."

I began building a bedroom on the main floor the next day. The construction was a modern day barn-raising with a fishing buddy, Ed Weisman, leading a team of volunteers. Everyone pitched in, donating their labor. Some afternoons looked like a block party. I supplied the beer and food. They supplied the muscle. I designed my room with beautiful skylights, French doors and huge triangular shaped windows.

So many patients I met wound up spending large amounts of time in bed. I assumed that was normal and I planned for that time.

I told everyone, "If ALS is going to keep me indoors and bedridden, then I will bring the outdoors inside."

The room was on a cement slab. Because of this, the addition could not be air-conditioned using ductwork from the basement. For years, I endured an oppressive, hot, sun-drenched bedroom. For a while, I made do with fans to shorten the sleepless summer nights. Now, more paralyzed from advancing ALS and no longer able to adjust to the heat, I was desperate. I could not survive another stifling summer in that room.

A chance question to a friend about new ductless AC units began a chain of events leading to an improbable ending, one topping the best Hollywood script because it was true. Someone made a call to a local HVAC firm, Soundview AC and Heating. The owner showed up at my house and scouted out the situation. Without any discussion, he proposed a simple solution to rescue me.

He had the same confidence as a modern day 'Can Do' cavalry soldier.

"A ductless heat pump unit will do the trick. I will put one in for you," he said with blithe.

I did not have that kind of money lying around. Before making such a decision, I would normally research units and compare prices. I didn't even ask this guy to come and look at the room. I timidly asked about the cost.

"Umm, how much is this gonna cost?"

"Nothing, I am giving it to you for free." was his answer.

"W H A T?" I uttered.

He explained the equipment was a demonstrator from the manufacturer. "I want to use it here." He also told me, "I will install it and coordinate the electrical work at no cost."

"I ah, I err," I could not find words. I was in shock. I managed to cough out, "Thank you, John."

Never would I, or could I, have thought this would be the ending to my sleepless nights.

Good guys in white hats do exist. Bad stories do have happy endings. . Improbable events happen. Miracles are real.

I kept saying, "Thank you and God bless you."

"You are welcome. You do good work for so many people. I want to help you." John said.

"Your great kindness will be paid forward in ways you will never know." I promised. "The next time you are surfing TV channels and an old Western is on, take a moment to watch some of it."

I told him.

"Okay….?" His voice trailing off. He looked at me not knowing where the hell I was going with this.

I said, "When the good guy appears and saves the day, I want you to smile. It is you on screen John. It will be like looking in the mirror. You are the guy in the white hat!"

The lesson in this was 'Good guys' are all around us. The help they provide comes in every imaginable form. It comes sometimes when we are most desperate.

Celebrating Hope

Hope is the most powerful force we possess. With it, mountains are moved and miracles are realized. I once read, "Hope will never leave you, it is you who will abandon it!"

When I received the long awaited telephone call that Columbus Day from my doctor who delivered the devastating diagnosis, I plunged into a dark, frightening world.
Medicine offered nothing.
The prognosis was bone-chillingly grim. The advice given to me "Put your life in order."
Sound advice according to most since ALS is considered hopeless.
Patients are expected to die within a few years of diagnosis.

I turned to my family, my friends and my faith.
They were my reservoir of strength.
Quietly, I held fast to a glimmering feeling deep within me. I hoped. There was no plan, or expectation. I had no vision of the future. I did not expect a cure. All I had was an indefinable but unshakeable

sense of hope. Though afraid, I took each day as it
came, considering it a gift. Over nine thousand, five
hundred days later,
each day continues to be one.

Tuesday begins my 27th year of living with ALS.
I celebrated my anniversary of living with good
friends, delicious food and a glorious setting at the
Cowfish restaurant on Shinnecock Bay.
Life poses great challenges but is precious and worth
living, even with the struggle.
Although now 69, totally disabled and ventilator
dependent,
I continue to hope, for God is indeed good.

I hope for my wife. I hope for my children and
grandchild.
I hope for the wonderful people who care for me
and those who care for others.
I hope for patients newly diagnosed. I hope for the
dedicated researchers toiling for cures.

My last hope I saved for all of you who read this
book.
Remember, it is people who abandon hope. It will
never abandon you.
It has been at my side this entire remarkable journey.
I hope it accompanies you.

The lesson I learned from this was to find reasons to hope from every day things. It is the fuel that propels you to continue.

Giving Thanks

At Thanksgiving, everyone reflects on blessings. I wrote about things many take for granted. They are the simple things we overlook that bring life alive.

I am grateful that my eyes opened this morning,
for I have been blessed with life.

I am grateful for my wife lying here, kids about in the world,
a delightful grandson,
for I have been blessed with family.

I am grateful for azure sky and white puffy clouds dancing
in skylights overhead,
for I have been blessed to see.

I am grateful for the beaming yellow sunrays warming my
cheek,
for I have been blessed to feel.

I am grateful for the aroma of brewing morning coffee waft-
ing through the air,
for I have been blessed to smell.

I am grateful for the creamy butter and sweet maple syrup
on my waffles,
for I have been blessed to taste.

I am grateful for the bluejay garishly squawking from the
bird feeder,
for I have been blessed to hear.

I am grateful for the skill to write this poem,
for I have been blessed to create and think.

I am grateful for all those who help and show concern about
me,
for I have been blessed with friendship.

I am grateful for amazing intellects who invented incredible
technology,
**For through them, I have been blessed with extended
living.**

I am grateful for the insightful and curious investigators
researching the causes of ALS,
for I am blessed with optimism of a cure.

I am grateful for the men and women devoting lives in service to others,
for I have been blessed with good care.

I am grateful for the generous business support of my life's
work finding a cure,

for I have been blessed knowing my disease has funds for
research.

I am grateful for all of the various ALS groups,
for they are organizing and fighting so I may live.

I am grateful for everything that I have endured,
for I have been blessed with purposeful living.

Finally, I am grateful to give thanks to God,
for I have been blessed with faith.

Even in this imperfect world, I will go to sleep this evening
and be at peace,
for I have been blessed with joy and live with hope.

The lesson in this was recognizing the wonderful blessings we have beyond the obvious. Give thanks for the every-
day things and the people who spend their lives working on
our behalf.

Dr. Seuss On Some Every Day Crap

After a rough week of hoyering, my behind was raw with abrasion from the straps. My skin ached with tenderness. Sitting on the bowl one time, it occurred to me how lucky someone was who just walked and sat down on the toilet. I wrote this poem as a result of that thought.

I don't like this, not one little bit,
It's a terrible way to go take a shit.
It is not fun, surely it is not,
Wish I could run. Run from this spot.

Who would think a trip to the bowl,
Could be so tough, taking a toll?
You won't like it if it happens to you,
'Cause it will leave your hiney sore and blue.

Getting to the toilet is no easy thing.
Using a gadget they call a hoyer sling.
I must be hoisted so high in the air,
That the whole thing takes the greatest of care.

Next time your bowels you want to please,
Head to the toilet with plenty of ease.
Go on, answer the call.
Sit, relax have a ball.

As you contemplate upon your throne,
Just muse over *the problems you own.*
And, don't think taking a crap is yucky,
The simple truth is, *you are damn lucky!*

The lesson in this was the ability to perform the most simple and basic functions of life are absolute blessings. These abilities and functions must never be taken for granted.

Part Two

Tales From The Road and The Lessons They Taught

Tell It To The Judge!

I grew up in the turbulent '60s. It was a time of tremendous social upheaval. The decade altered America forever. The agents of this change were activists leading protests and marches. I witnessed close up the power of people uniting for a change and individuals making a difference.

Dr. Martin Luther King and his epic struggle to gain equal rights for African-Americans and every citizen shaped my world. Seared into my mind are images of gushing fire hoses knocking protesters down, store boycotts, freedom riders and the March on Washington. Mass gatherings at parks, waterways, forests and factories birthed the environmental movement. The recent photographs sent back to earth from the astronauts changed our view of our fragile and isolated planet. Attention focused on "spaceship earth," a term used to describe the new perspective of our planet traveling through the universe. Angry confrontations, flag burnings, University shut downs with chants of, "Hell no I won't go" rocked the nation. Each night's news broadcast of body counts and military coffins brought the brutal war into the living rooms of America.

During my senior year in college, the anti-war protests reached a trigger point. On April 30, 1970, President Nixon ordered the bombing of Cambodia, a major expansion of the war. An estimated four million high school and college students walked out of classes in a massive protest. The next day Ohio State University erupted in violent demonstrations. By May 4, the situation was out of control. Authorities called in the Ohio National Guard to campus. They carried automatic weapons with live ammunition to break up a protest of kids. At noon, the massacre of innocent, unarmed college students began. In all, 29 students were wounded and four killed.

The next day protesters descended on my college, Fredonia State University of New York, and took it over forcing it to close. I was off campus doing my student teaching. I returned to campus and marched with thousands of fellow protesters through the town. That weekend, many of us went 50 miles northward to Buffalo. A huge number of students from the University of Buffalo and surrounding colleges took over a main thoroughfare of the city, Bailey Avenue. They built barricades and burned furniture. Nervous police stood on the perimeter areas. It was a surreal scene. Frightened by the violence the authorities inflicted on students at Kent State, I feared for my safety. As ominous as that danger felt, it paled to what the military faced 8,000 miles across the ocean. Our protests helped to an end the derisive Vietnam War.

Throngs of women burning their bras demanded gender equality in business, society and politics. The playing field, while still not level, is more even today because of those pioneers. These were epic events that molded my mind.

For me, the remarkable results of these movements underscored the power of choosing to make a difference. The activists of those movements did more than complain about these wrongs; rather they opted to fight for change. This activism formed a model in my subconscious. I followed this model 40 years later.

Like most, when diagnosed, I did not know much about this disease. The more I learned the more I realized the disease needed awareness. Patients died by the thousands every year and few people knew about the disease. The number diagnosed with ALS is similar to Multiple Sclerosis. The latter is widely known and ALS is not. MS patients live for decades, forming a large core of supporters. By comparison, ALS claims patients so fast that few live long enough to rally a community of supporters. There were no organized, effective advocacy efforts at the time of my diagnosis in 1993.

Year after year, ALS continued unabated. There remained no outcry, no public pressure for research. Patients languished, often shut away in back rooms of nursing homes, helpless and hopeless. Early on, it became apparent I had a slow progression. It seemed I would escape the awful prognosis. I received a precious gift. I had more time to live.

"How would I use it?" I asked aloud.

One fall morning in 1997 at the start of a new school term, a colleague from my Dickinson Ave. School, Pam Cirasole, happened to be at the teacher mailboxes in the office at work the same time I was. Standing behind me, she watched as I struggled to open a sealed envelope from my mailbox. I battled mighty against its unyielding gum seal. ALS rendered the simple task of opening a plain envelope nearly impossible. My weakened fingers and useless arms were a poor match for strong business envelope made to survive a perilous journey in the US mail.

Seeing my difficulty, she interrupted me.

"Do you need a hand with that, Chris?" she asked.

"No thanks, I almost have it." I smiled.

I returned to the defiant envelope and continued my assault. Plopping one hand on top to hold it, I managed to get a fingernail under the flap. I pushed my entire finger in and loosened the seal a fraction. After numerous attempts, I breached the seal and overcame the remaining resistance. Like spoils of war, I pulled out the letter in triumph and read it. Pam watched the entire episode and vowed in silence.

"I will help him some way!" she swore.

In late October, she organized her music department throughout the Northport E. Northport School district to produce a fundraiser for ALS. The administration threw their support behind her project. They provided a school auditorium. The custodial staff donated their services. Flutists, guitarists, pianists, singers and brass players, all music teachers in the district, joined her to support my cause. This was the first ALS event held for me. Friends and family came. It was a packed house.

At the end, I took the stage to give my thanks. A week before the event, I broke my leg resulting in a soft cast. Already challenged to walk, I now staggered and limped across the stage.

"I am standing before you because I CAN!" I told the audience half-joking.

First, I expressed my appreciation to Pam and the performers as well as the administration. Then, I used the opportunity to announce a crazy dream. Although I mulled it over in my mind for months, I never said anything in public before. Pumped up by the exuberant moment, I suspended judgment and blurted it out.

"I am riding my wheelchair to Washington DC in the May for ALS awareness month."

The audience roared in approval and cheered. Now, I needed to back up the bravado with action. May was just seven months away.

Yankee Stadium is ground zero for the baseball world. Many consider the ballpark sacred ground. Any awareness campaign about ALS originating in the New York area had to include the stadium. The question for me was, how could I get their attention and secure permission to begin my Ride there?

I had to start the Ride to Washington from the place where Gehrig played and delivered his memorable farewell. There were no options. The Yankee organization is one of the most storied in the universe. I soon discovered gaining access to them was beyond hard.

Initially, I contacted their Community Relations Department. I wrote an impassioned plea detailing my diagnosis with ALS and my desire to cure the disease. The disease took their beloved Iron Horse, so I was optimistic. I presented my plan to ride from the Stadium to Washington spreading awareness. I awaited their reply of support for my project with guarded confidence.

I waited. I did not factor the Yankees getting scores of worthy requests for assistance every day. My letter sat under the pile of pleas. Weeks passed. In the absence of approval, planning continued on other fronts. I got my students and school involved. We researched routes and wrote letters. They designed tee shirts. The entire school community gave me overwhelming support. Parents stepped forward to offer help and words of encouragement. Dickinson Avenue Elementary became the hub for the developing ALS Ride for Life.

I learned that one of my student's mother lost her great aunt to ALS. One afternoon, Yvonne Giovinico came to school to pick up her daughter, Kristina. I saw the two of them standing and said hello. We wound up talking about the Ride, which by now was the buzz of the building.

"Hello Mr. Pendergast," she said. "I lost my aunt and would love to help."

"I don't have an exact plan. I need help figuring it all out." I told her.

"My family and I will help whatever way we can." she assured.

She joined a nucleus of key supporters helping me organize the Ride throughout the winter, often around her dining room table as we ate delicious spaghetti. Her husband, Frank, worked as a construction manager at the reconstruction of the Bronx County Courthouse building. As he roamed the building during construction, he met many employees. One person proved important: Nancy Vendetti, a secretary for some judges.

She and Frank often exchanged small talk. She shared the recent loss of her father to ALS. Right away Frank told her about his wife's work with this teacher. He mentioned the Ride to D.C. starting at the Stadium. A typical New Yorker, impatient and blunt, he then lambasted the Yankees silence on my request.

"Those bums won't even answer him," he complained.

Nancy's mind raced. She wanted to fight back in her dad's honor and formed a plan. A well- known New York State Supreme Court Judge, Howard Silver, came to mind. She knew his wife, Bea, was battling ALS. She also knew he was a huge Yankee fan.

The next day she spoke with the judge. She asked him if he would intercede with the Yankees on behalf of Bea and all PALS.

"They need help to get Yankee support for the Ride. Will you please make a call for them Judge?" she asked.

"I will be happy to assist," he replied.

He called Debbie Tyman, Community Affairs Coordinator for the Yankees. She did not return his call. After several days without an answer, he called back. This time Debbie responded.

"Hello Judge, how can I help you?" she asked.

"You can start by answering me the first time I telephone you!" he pronounced as if speaking to someone appearing in his courtroom.

"Yes, Judge!"

This certainly got her attention and set the stage for his request to assist a Lou Gehrig's patient planning a trip to Washington beginning at the Stadium. He pled his case and my fate rested in Debbie's hands. Within a couple of days, I received a phone call from the Yankees.

"Your request has been approved," the spokesperson said.

Our crusade for awareness would begin where Lou Gehrig walked, and played for 17 years. By the February thaw, things were heating up with the Ride planning. We had the starting point.

On a sunny day in May to begin our first Ride in 1998, we assembled in front of the nine- story Bronx County Court building, an area aptly named Lou Gehrig Plaza. The Plaza opened in the 1930s, the heyday of the Gehrig era. Sitting atop a high rock outcropping, Gehrig Plaza dominated the area. A quarter mile down the wide Concourse Boulevard stood Yankee Stadium.

Bea Silver, the judge's wife, along with several other patients, departed the Plaza in various motorized mobility devices and headed to the Stadium the morning the first Ride began. Frank emceed a small send-off ceremony in a city park opposite the Stadium. We paid homage to the legend, prayed for PALS and for a cure. The Bronx Borough President Fernando Ferrer delivered the keynote speech and closed with wishing us good luck. We went across the street and volunteers stretched a blue ribbon across the sidewalk at the Yankee Press Gate.

Everyone counted down, "10, 9, 8, 7, 6, 5, 4, 3, 2, 1,"

"Let the Ride begin!" Frank shouted. A group cut the ribbon and we were off.

The other patients left. Fernando Tedesco, another ALS patient from my support group and I turned towards the George Washington Bridge and points south.

Bea died not too long after. Her battle was sadly on target for average survival. Thanks to her husband, Judge Silver, her fight continues today, decades after her death.

The ALS Ride for Life maintains a close relationship with the Yankees and PALS from the Ride have appeared on home plate twenty times. Debbie Tyman is one of our closest supporters.

The Yankee connection all started with a child's concern for her teacher, her empathetic mother, her gregarious father and a civil servant working in a courthouse who was willing to "tell it to the judge." Each was willing to make a difference. Each was willing to share my dream.

The lesson I learned from this was the value of having someone open the door. Unfortunately, no matter the importance or worthwhile the cause, reality is the plea for help gets buried under a slew of others. Success often depends on who you know and a good measure of luck. Open doors whenever you get the opportunity.

The Brotherhood of Blue

I was a latch key kid before the term came into popular use. My Grandmother watched me when we lived together in Mineola. My youngest aunt, Elizabeth, married right after high school. I was four years old yet remember the commotion at our house the day of the wedding. I spent a good amount of time with my aunt and her new husband, Bob. My uncle became a police officer and they raised their family on Long Island, near my home.

In the summer of 1954, we moved to Mt. Sinai to be near Port Jefferson's Wharton Memorial School, a residential facility for children with polio and other developmental problems where my older brother Tom went to live. He suffered a brain injury at birth leaving him with developmental deficits. My mom had to continue working and farmed me out to relatives during school vacations. Many of those times were spent with Aunt Elizabeth and her family.

Growing up, my relationship with my Uncle Bob was good, although slightly distant. Typical of many police from his generation, he was austere and authoritative. A story spinner, he loved telling jokes. He drank Rheingold beer as we watched NY Ranger Hockey and Yankee baseball games on TV. I loved him but my young mind always felt uneasy around him because he was so direct, strict and authoritarian

—there was no softness. Our families grew old together and I remained tight with them and their six children. My diagnosis brought out a flood of support from their family. Much more was to come.

I already mentioned my frustration at the lack of understanding about ALS and the low levels of research. It is obvious why I was happy announcing my plan to organize a Ride to Washington at Pam's concert. Now the work began. I knew I needed the cooperation of police along the route. I worried the departments would reject the nutty idea of riding my wheelchair down their streets. I reached out to my uncle for help organizing my first Ride and enlisted him to shoulder the task of getting the police to agree. I reasoned a brother officer asking for help to save his dying nephew seemed more effective than a request from a private citizen.

"Uncle Bob, I have a crazy idea I want to run by you."

"I am listening. Go on," he said. I laid out my plan.

"Of course!" he answered without hesitation. "I'd be proud to do it for you." So much for the austere memory of old Uncle Bob. He went to work right away.

"Tell me again about plans for Trenton," or some other city he would excitedly ask each time he got another return call from his inquiry.

"Okay, Uncle Bob," and I would provide the general details minus a specific route. He was successful and got all the larger-known departments to sign on. The Ride was in motion.

When spring arrived, we embarked on our 14-day journey to the Capitol. Several days in, we approached Philadelphia from the northwest through the rolling hills of Bucks County.

Forests interspersed with small fields surrounded the single lane road we traveled. Residences were scattered along the curving route. We made steady progress, covering a mile every ten or twelve minutes.

In those days, Google Maps did not exist. It was not easy to identify the police jurisdictions along our journey and we missed many of the small ones in unincorporated areas. The police "handed" me off to the next adjoining department even if we didn't contact them ahead of time. The hand offs made it possible to get each agency's cooperation, even if they were unaware.

One police department in the area was particularly small. The officer handled the duty solo. Five miles into his escort, the traffic began accumulating. Each curve we rounded allowed me to look backward. Cars and pick-ups stretched all the way back to the next bend. I felt guilty causing an unnecessary traffic jam.

"Maybe we should pull off at the next wide point and allow traffic to pass." I relayed up to the police officer. He stopped the squad car in the road and came back to talk.

"You have permission to do this. This is your road for the moment. There are other ways for the cars to get around us," he said to me without sympathy for the motorists. "How about you? Are you doing okay?" shifting the focus to my well-being.

"I am thanks. This is a beautiful section and I am enjoying it. Your support and understanding are fantastic," I said.

"Well then, let's get going." He turned and headed back to his patrol car.

Back on the road again, I mulled over his comment. Disabled people are almost always a second thought. We wait practically all the time. It is rare we come first. Here, I thought, the officer made us the priority and made the traffic wait. It was an unusual experience for me—one that made me uncomfortable at first. The more I thought, the more I welcomed his decision. His action had a powerful impact. Finally, without hesitation, the disabled went to the front of the line!

In an hour or two, we reached the end of the jurisdiction and did the hand off. The next department was waiting and we pulled over to make the switch. I signaled my team to get a tee shirt for the departing police officer and one for his chief.

"You moved me with your decision to prioritize the Ride. I felt validated. It motivated me to persevere in the hard times to come. God bless you. Please accept this tee shirt." I presented it to him.

"I understand what this means. It was my privilege and honor, sir. I wish you the best. I hope you find a cure soon. Thank you for doing this. God bless YOU!" Smiling, he took the shirts.

Then, he dropped a bombshell. He confessed, "My Uncle died from ALS not too long ago."

He held the shirts tight, pivoted and walked off. The next department was waiting. I became preoccupied talking with the next escort. By the time we finished the conference, the officer was gone. I never got an opportunity to express my thoughts and appreciation for his kindness.

I always wait in the rear of the line of wheelchairs for one reason or another. I do not push to be first. I am willing to wait. Tucked in rural Pennsylvania, miles from anywhere on a quiet afternoon, a police officer affected me as few have done. He chose me over the din and clamor. He affirmed my value by putting me first.

"The last shall be first and the first shall be last." Matthew 20:16

In a mysterious way, a brotherhood of blue came full circle: Two uncles: one a cop, one a patient, and two nephews: one a cop, the other, a patient. The two cops linked by family and disease.

Austere no more.

Police are the unsung heroes of the Ride. Without their expert escorts, the Ride as we know it would not exist. In the most trying of circumstances, they safely navigate a group of wheelchairs along with a gaggle of supporters through every conceivable road and traffic situation whether rain or shine.

The police family is not immune to ALS. In the first support group my wife attended, she met the wife of a police officer from Nassau County with ALS. When Christine returned the next month, he was dead. SCPD had Neil Keating. NYPD officer, Lenny Crawford, died from it. The Freeport Police suffered the loss of its Union President and popular officer, Jack Lundergan. Recently, the Lynbrook Department commander, Ron Fleury, died. The list goes on and on.

When they assist the Ride, they are serving fallen brothers as well. I salute them for their help.

The lesson I learned from this was authority figures maintain a necessary professional persona but beneath that façade resides a compassionate human being. Police officers are a prime example.

Necessity Is the Mother of Invention

The Ride pieces were coming together. The next obstacle on the plans revolved around the actual route. At this point, all I had was a dream. I needed a pathway to reach it. Someone must drive and help me scout out a route. I asked Christine for help and she didn't want to do it.

The more I mentioned the Ride to my wife, the more she blew me off causing a big strain on our relationship. It was not until much later I found out the reason.

"I was worried," she confessed. "I hoped if I ignored you long enough you would get tired and drop the whole crazy idea!"

I always said to her, "I would rather be killed fighting it than by it!"

Since January, I wanted to start laying out the detailed route for the trip. She ignored repeated requests to spend a few weekends with me driving the proposed roadways. By February discouraged but determined, I sought alternatives. Most of my friends were either married with children or otherwise committed.

I looked around. No one in my inner circle seemed available. I felt too intimidated to ask those who possibly would be

159

able to help. I suppose I did not feel worthy of their sacrifice. My hunt for help seemed like the hit song of the Oscar winning movie from the 70's, *The Urban Cowboy*: "I was looking for help in all the wrong places."

There was a friend from work, an excellent classroom teacher that I held in high regard. She was a confidant of sorts. She had a similar, child-centered philosophy of teaching. She embraced the same experiential approach to teaching and was a cleansing breath of fresh air from many of the teachers with whom I interacted. My salvation to my Ride dilemma was right in front of me.

Jane Flood taught in Dickinson Avenue School. Early in her career, she left teaching to raise her family. Now divorced and children grown, she did not have the obligations that prevented others from helping.

One frustrated Thursday night after another "no" from my concerned wife, I phoned Jane with a hair-brained request. I got an answering machine.

"Will you drive me to Washington this weekend?" My question was abrupt.

Soon after, she called back from a local Irish pub with her shocking answer.

"I'm ready! My friend and I will be there," she yelled over the noisy bar background.

Before breakfast Saturday morning Jane, John and I set off with an armful of maps, note pads and plenty of sharpened pencils. For the next two weekends, we drove back and forth between Long Island and New Jersey. We snaked our way beyond points south of the George Washington Bridge searching for a route.

I had no idea what I was doing. I didn't realize this ride was not so different from other special memorial runs or bicycle trips going to Washington. The entire time I was looking for a route I could travel alone without any outside assistance. I picked a proposed route from the map ahead of time and we would test them. Often they ended with an impassable obstacle.

"Damn, I'll never be able to get around that. We gotta turn around and try something else," I would say in disappointment.

"Great planning Chris," Jane ribbed me with her biting wit.

"Never mind, just write down the mile point." I'd shoot back. Then I would blast the numbers too fast for her write down.

"Wait, slow down," she'd protest.

"Well, if you would pay attention and not be commenting so much, you would be ready." I needled her right back.

It was frustrating and progress was slow. Mile by mile we inched our way down, Jane did her best to scribble the road names and distances that rolled off my tongue in rapid order. By the second weekend, Jersey route was complete. The proof of concept was established. We were on the way to a successful, detailed route for the whole trip.

I was ready to begin other phases of planning, scheduling. Christine began to accept the reality of my trip. The crazy idea she hoped I would drop was in fact, happening.

A proverb says 'necessity is the mother of invention'. The Ride for Life was born out of necessity to address the deplorable state of ALS awareness and advocacy. This time however, necessity was a midwife. Jane is the real mother of the Ride for Life.

Congratulations Jane. You gave birth to a beautiful baby.

The lesson I learned from this was be brave and don't let insecurity and fear of rejection interfere with your dreams. Ask and you shall receive.

Leader(s) of the Pack

Leaders emerge during a time of need. As the Ride moved through different stages, it depended on many volunteers for their leadership to guide the Ride. One of the first, Martin Haley, was my Suffolk County Legislator. He found out about my advocacy work from Ray Manzoni, a hometown friend who knew of my beginning attempts at bringing awareness and fundraising.

"I want the County to recognize you for your outstanding work in the ALS community," Haley said. I spoke with him to get specifics.

"Martin, can the proclamation recognize my school district rather than me because they were at the heart of the much of my efforts?"

"Of course," he answered.

The district superintendent was Dr. William Brosnan. He was a strong supporter of my pioneering classroom programs and continued this with my advocacy work. Without his pivotal approval, the up-coming Ride would be dead in its tracks. He was the obvious choice to accept the accolade for the district from the County Legislature. I thought it would bind him tightly to the Ride.

"Dr. Brosnan, the County is honoring the District and me for the Advocacy work being done. Will you accept the proclamation at a public session of the Legislature?" I asked.

"It would be an honor, Chris. I'm happy to go with you, the students and accept."

I brought my class to the morning session, along with some parents and my family. Many students were working on the Ride plans. Mr. Haley introduced me and Dr. Bill Brosnan. He presented the proclamation and both Brosnan and I gave our thanks. Students smiled for photos with the Legislature. Parents lined up to snap pictures with their elected representative.

After everything ended, my boss pulled me aside.

"Thanks for including the District and students with your honor," he continued talking, "Whatever else I can do to help don't hesitate to ask."

Little did he know he just opened ALS's equivalent of Pandora's Box.

With the logistical plans moving along, I turned my attention to figuring out my teaching schedule and getting released time to go on the Ride. I made an appointment to meet with the assistant superintendent for personnel. I requested permission to have a two-week leave and use my accumulated sick day benefit to enable my pay to continue. He listened with patience and made notes.

"I will consider it. Give me some time to look into this, Chris. I will let you know in a few days."

I left the meeting with an optimistic feeling. True to his word, he sent a response through interoffice mail.

"Good luck, Chris. You do not have to deplete your sick days. Your salary will continue," his memo stated.

"Wow!" I exclaimed. The memo was more support than I anticipated. A full leave without using my sick days, "Yahoo!" I moved to the next issues.

How would I pay all the expense? The hotels, food, supplies and equipment expenses were way too much for me to pay. How would I get a wheelchair down there? I was doing this to help the ALS community, not personal gain. I needed support.

I approached the Suffolk chapter of the Muscular Dystrophy Association and the ALS Association of Greater New York. I prepared a budget to cover basic expenses and asked for a sponsorship. I was disappointed when the MDA flat out refused.

"The event involved overlapping chapter jurisdictions and that makes sponsoring impossible," they explained. "Each chapter is independent and has their own budget," was the justification they gave. They threw in, "Safety is a concern, too." They worry about me getting hurt. What a joke! I'm dying....

My last hope was the newly formed New York chapter of the ALS Association. Dorine Gordon, chapter President, lost her father to ALS. She was more receptive to my request. We already worked on several fundraising campaigns. She knew my ability to organize and deliver.

"We will give a grant for up to $10,000 to cover Ride costs," she said. In addition, she offered their logistical support. "We will assist with hotels, food and mobile phones (at that time an expensive item)," she told me. To start with, I received a used handicapped van from the loaner program. The van was a major reduction in the cost of the Ride.

I set the timing of the Ride so we would arrive in Washington DC to coordinate with National Advocacy Day on The Hill. This was the first gathering of ALS patients and their supporters. The ALS Association organized this important convening of advocates to make a unified effort to influence Congress. The partnership between ALSA GNY and my journey promised to be a win for both. Most important, it was a win for the ALS community. The progressive leadership provided by Dorine has left a tremendous legacy. The Ride owes it start in large part to her. The support she gave produced high dividends over the years. Our organization has given well over one million dollars in funding for the ALS Association. They are our highest grantee.

With these logistical items resolved, one gaping hole remained in our plans. Who will comprise my volunteers on the Ride itself? Who would help me on the road? Christine would be working. Who would make the executive decisions, serve as the contact point and handle the endless minutia to come while on the road?

The Superintendent visited our school soon after the Proclamation ceremony. I happened to be in the office when he arrived. Dr. Burns greeted him. In an unplanned encounter, we all chatted a bit about the ceremony. The topic switched to Ride planning. Both men reiterated their desire to help.

"Thanks, I am grateful for all you both have done already!" I said. "I will be certain to let you know if I need anything."

The physical education teacher was sitting in the office waiting on another matter. Charlie Catania and I spoke little.

Our schedules did not overlap and we almost never saw one another in the building. He ran after-school programs that occupied him at the end of the day, the time I was available. We traveled in different circles. As a result, we knew almost nothing about each other.

He floored me when he said, "Chris, I'm interested in helping you too. Is there anything you need?"

A humorous expression developed at the Ride regarding volunteers. Each newbie receives a warning.

"Be very careful about what you say to Chris, for you'll be sorry!"

The admonition concerned getting too close to the 'event horizon,' a term to describe the edge of a Black Hole. If you reach this horizon, gravity will suck you down into the hole, never to emerge. You vanish to the outside world. Even light cannot escape once it enters the hole. Charlie went too close. It drew him into a Ride Black Hole. His life changed forever. Mine did as well.

Charlie received the same leave conditions as me. He grew to be an integral component of each ALS Ride. No other person played a more pivotal role leading the Ride. He earned the nickname "St. Charles" because of his devotion and commitment to the patients and Ride. He became a legend in Northport for his extensive Ride work. The next six years he led us on successful Rides. His daughter, Katie, attended Dickinson and was a fabulous Habitat Helper. She joined her Dad on Friday and became a weekend wheelchair jockey, whipping around hotel parking lots at day's end. She and my son were close in age. For years, the two came down to work. They drove the wheelchairs from the trailer to the charging room in the hotel. They gathered patients' chairs at the end of the night to charge them. They were so helpful. On the road, they accompanied PALS and assisted however needed.

A week into the first Ride, Nancy Venditti, the secretary from the Bronx Supreme Court, contacted us several days into the Ride. She announced there was a surprise waiting for us back at the hotel in Maryland. Her brother, Bob Cauttero worked on something for the Ride. He was a self-admitted computer geek. Posting photos was not common back before Facebook and other social media websites made it easy. Bob used his technical skills and delighted everyone by posting the Ride photos online.

The Ride was able to go national at a time when there was little activism available across the country. His contributions were groundbreaking. Patients across the country saw the advocacy efforts on their behalf. It opened a new outlet to push for change. It inspired them. An era of national organizing was beginning.

Bob's support evolved, and when we incorporated a year later, he served as Vice President. Nancy served as our first Secretary. Both pushed hard to implement patient service. I wanted to emphasize researching a cure to spare another family from this heartache. Seeking compromise, we created a novel nursing assistance program, which Nancy supervised for several years. It was the first nursing program offered across the country to help PALS and their families.

When we conduct the Ride, patients are supposed to participate on the Ride in a 'self-contained' condition. This meant they should be independent and have their own support team. Rarely did that happen. In good conscience, I could not exclude a dying patient an opportunity to participate because family or friends were unable to assist them on the road. Yet, we lacked the staff to help them. Thank God, a wonderful man who recently retired from administration in the district came from out of the blue to volunteer Larry McNally.

Dr. Larry McNally was part of the 'Driving Chris' team organized by my caring building principal, Gary. When my driving to work reached a questionable level, I continued anyway unable to accept the reality of my progression. Concerned for my safety and for the surrounding motorists, Gary put out a secret notice.

"I am requesting volunteers to drive Chris to and from work each day-an hour each way," he said in a letter sent throughout the entire district.

When he organized it and had 50 drivers scheduled, he called me in his office.

"Chris, sit down, I have something to discuss." he began.

He laid out his plan. Fellow teachers, custodians, teacher aides, kitchen workers, administrators, parents and a school board member signed up to drive me back and forth each day. For those living in the Northport area, it was a two-hour commitment.

"Gary, I don't know what to say. I am overwhelmed. I am humbled." I choked up. My insecurities always force me to under value my worth. I was surprised so many held me in this high regard.

During my last three years, I taught part time because state law required I exhaust my sick time before applying for disability. Without these wonderful volunteer drivers, my career and advocacy would have grinded to a halt. Once again, the loving kindness of others saved me.

Larry McNally was one of the drivers. We loved our rides together. He was a well-educated, articulate and engaging man committed to helping others, a reflection of his psychologist training. We formed a strong bond of friendship and respect. It came as no surprise; Larry became the patient coordinator for the Ride. He provided invaluable services for patients attending each Ride for many years, even after he moved to Florida. He continues to this day, although in a more limited role.

The last of these leaders to recognize is my union President, Bill Hall. He was a silent guiding light. There were numerous issues related to my work. He provided advice to help me steer though the juggernaut of employment matters. He instilled confidence and encouraged me when I wavered. Bill organized a union sponsored kickoff, the forerunner of our current and successful Honoree Recognition Benefit.

I told Bill, "You believed in me before I believed in myself! If you didn't have that faith in me, I am not certain where my journey would have ended. Thank you for seeing something in me before I saw it."

A disproportionate number of leaders of the ALS Ride for Life came from the Northport School community. The brilliant mathematician, Edward Lorenz, demonstrated beyond a doubt, that a butterfly's wing movement effects a tornado weeks later. Small things that seem of minor importance produce significant consequences later.

It is hard to comprehend the impact of this community on the lives of thousands of ALS patients and their families. The extraordinary research conducted due to these people altered the course of ALS science. They have improved the lives of hundreds of ALS patients. Thousands of students and adults know about the Long Island Ride. Millions of Americans have learned about ALS because of their actions.

It was a remarkable confluence of people, location and time. They were the leaders of the pack.

The lesson I learned from this was your greatest allies are often surrounding you. Live a life defined by integrity and kindness. When you need leaders to champion your mission, they will rise around you.

Jumpers

"Indescribable," I said.

It is the only one way I *can* describe the excitement. We assembled at Gehrig's Plaza, the NYS Supreme Court complex in the Bronx for the first Ride in 1998. It was electrifying. The massive Greco-Roman building standing atop a rise of land north of the Harlem River made an impressive backdrop. With its commanding view of the south Bronx and Yankee Stadium a short distance away, it was the perfect start for the first day of the inaugural Ride for Life to Washington DC, an odyssey leading to adventures and destinations unknown.

Several other patients and I lined up our machines facing south on the Grand Concourse, a major thoroughfare running the length of the Borough. The road shot straight through the heart of the South Bronx. Down the gentle slope near the river was Yankee Stadium. This fabled borough of the city had seen better economic days. The neighborhood was riddled with poverty and those expressions were evident everywhere.

I shouted, "Gentlemen, start your engines!"

With shouts of good luck, we were off. Our disability scooters and wheelchairs cruised along at an easy gait. A couple of bicyclists, including my seventh-grade son, accompanied the patients as we proceeded behind the phalanx of police who were escorting us. Amid the commotion, which defines an urban area, the odd caravan still managed to raise eyebrows.

After an emotional stop at the old Yankee Stadium, we left the Bronx. We headed over the Harlem River on the McCombs Dam Bridge and into upper Manhattan. Our first day on the Ride was through New York City, across the mighty Hudson and down northern New Jersey.

It seemed ironic. Washington Heights, our first area in Manhattan was Lou Gehrig's neighborhood. Long a melting pot, it was now boiling with vibrancy from recent Colombian, Dominican and other South American immigrants. Our public awareness campaign was in its infancy back in those days. We had no bilingual literature explaining ALS. I wondered what the people thought as they watched the police lead us through their community. The handicapped scooter I rode cost a few months' salary for some of them. Amid the poverty, I felt a bit uneasy, hoping they would understand our suffering. ALS knows no national boundaries. I am riding for all of them, even though they may not realize it.

Highway One is a special NYPD unit that specialized in public affairs, foreign dignitaries, parades and similar events. The detail serves all of the five boroughs. They did their job well and knew all the major thoroughfares of the City. They were not familiar with the local neighborhoods, which precincts serve. Since we traveled across the city, they escorted us.

Their massive, powerful and fast Harley Davidsons were a stark contrast to our slow-moving disability vehicles. As we inched toward the famous George Washington Bridge, various police units peeled off or joined. Police scooters threaded through the gnarled traffic. Motorcycles blocked intersections. The bicycle unit flanked our sides. We navigated some of the most congested urban streets in the country thanks to New York's finest. It was organized mayhem, yet they made it look easy.

My pre-trip planning identified the GW Bridge had pedestrian/bike paths both east and westbound. The Bridge was the one portal out of New York available to us. In the days before GPS, the road atlas showed the route and access to the bike path. Each of us were thrilled at the prospect of crossing suspended high above the Hudson on one of the most famous bridges in the world. The panorama promised to be breathtaking.

We rolled up near the bridge well behind schedule. Rather than being late morning, it was now mid-afternoon, and traffic was full blown. Our route, Broadway, ran right into US 1, the major artery linking the entire east coast. It claimed the entire lower six lanes of the Bridge while the upper Bridge was devoted to I-95. Our police escort was under enormous stress. Our safety was their primary goal. Ensuring the safety of wheelchair/scooters amidst the nightmare traffic, well-known impatient New Yorkers, racing cabbies, limos darting, delivery trucks, lumbering city buses and confused immigrant drivers was no easy task. At the same time, they had to keep the city's lifeblood flowing through its arteries. It was a balancing act worthy of a circus appearance. All that remained of their assignment was to get us across the highway and over to the bike path. Once we were on the bike path, it was a clear shot to Jersey. Their escort was almost complete.

The cops eased us onto US 1, bringing the already slow-moving traffic to a crawl. Rolling along at four miles an hour seems quick when sitting in the wheel chair or scooter, but a snail's pace behind the wheel of an automobile. The squad closed two approach lanes and confined us to the right lane. They allowed traffic to pass on the outside lane at a reduced speed.

The tall towers suspending the Bridge rose up straight into the sky in front of us. Sitting on the access road approaching the bridge was electrifying. The situation neared chaos. Cacophonous sounds rang out from every quarter: horns honked non-stop, truck air brakes belched, tires whined on the hot asphalt streets, taxi cabs squealed as they stopped and planes roared overhead. We pumped with adrenaline knowing that for once, we were putting ALS on the map. *THIS* was awareness! For once, this bastard disease did not have the upper hand.

All of a sudden, one of the police on the bicycle unit came over, shouting to us that we could not get across the westbound bike path on the north side of the bridge as planned. It had steps on the Jersey side that the wheelchairs could not do. So much for careful planning! One can only be as good as the tools used. Nowhere in any of the information did it indicate just one of the two bike paths was barrier free.

The ranking officer brought our procession to a halt right on the approach of the Bridge. When we stopped, so did the thousands of cars queued up behind us. We huddled in the road, like a football team on the goal line trying to move into the end zone. We had to back up and enter the southern path from a feeder road about three-eighths of a mile behind us. During the impromptu conference on US 1, the traffic backed up through the Bronx, making me think of the 1960s sitcom, *Car 54 Where Are You* jingle, which comically sung the same line.

It was another crazy day in New York. Behind us, the traffic was a solid wall for miles. Backing up was not an option. Going across the pathway was not an option. We could not abort the crossing and travel in our handicapped vehicles because they were ahead of us. It was an insane situation. The Sergeant made a decision to resolve the impasse and return traffic to its normal zaniness.

They wanted to shut down the entire upper westbound George Washington Bridge.

"But, we don't have jurisdiction," interjected one of the cops. "This is PA territory and they will NOT be happy."

It was true, NYPD jurisdiction ended at the Bridge. The Port Authority patrolled New York City's interstate bridges and tunnels. NYPD had no power to authorize our transit across the Bridge. As everywhere, policing agencies vigorously guard their turf.

The Ride was five hours old and already it appeared to face an unsolvable situation. In an ironic twist on the pun, "we could not cross that bridge once we came to it!"

"We are doing it," the senior officer announced. "By the time PA gets wind of it, we will be across!"

One man's decisive, proactive choice propelled the Ride forward. Onto the steel street of the bridge! We rode across in utter ecstasy. High above the Hudson, panoramic views on all sides, the ride was epic. Inbound traffic stopped with rubberneckers staring in disbelief at the site of a couple of paralyzed men sitting in scooters/wheelchairs tooling across the bridge. The unlikely scene made the evening news. It was a triumphant moment for ALS awareness.

As we neared the Jersey side, I shared my utter amazement with the sergeant.

"I will never forget this," I said. It was something that is not supposed to happen, even once in a lifetime.

"The George Washington Bridge never gets closed down like this. It is done only for crazy people and jumpers," he told me. I looked him straight in the eye and smiled.

"You got it half right, Sergeant. People tell me I *am* crazy for doing this trip," I told him, "But, I'm not gonna jump. I want to be around to see the ALS cure!" I announced.

That was 1998. I am still waiting.

The lesson I learned from this was that the best made plans go awry. Rather than become paralyzed with fear, effective people make bold, decisive decisions. Success or failure relies on such action. Don't shy from these opportunities.

Tale of Two Cities

Areas surrounding New York City such as the sections to the immediate west are one continuous sprawl of congestion. As you head southwest into New Jersey, the land opens. The rural land is broken by population centers every so often. Our route included some of both.

Both Princeton and Trenton are seats of power. One is the epitome of wealth and intellectual achievement. The other a government seat of power, the state capital. A mere ten miles separate the two. It might as well be an ocean because they are worlds apart. The opening lines of Charles Dicken's classic, "It was the best of times. It was the worst of times," well describes these two cities. One city is a flourishing center of the entitled. The other is choking with poverty, drugs and a failing, broken system. One thrives, one dies.

The Ride went through each of them. We selected Princeton to raise awareness and put a face on this neglected disease. A student at the University had a father battling ALS. We went there to visit her, tour the campus and dedicate the day to her dad. Out of all the prospective sources of research and technological development, there are few better places than Princeton University. To promote government support and spread awareness, we chose the state capital in Trenton.

"Now this is what I like," Fernando quipped referring to the Princeton area. "It's beautiful." The area contrasted the urban environment of the past days.

Roads outside Princeton were smooth, wide and clean. Nearing the town, the homes grew larger, lawns greener and neighborhoods prettier. The area had a quaint ambience. People walking on the sidewalks congested the downtown center. Attractive shops invited passers-by to enter. Customers filled boutiques and coffee shops. It appeared a perfect town to visit.

Traffic clogged the streets. Our slow police escort approached the middle of town. In time, everything seemed to change. Rude street pedestrians cut between the wheel-chairs and the police. So did motorists. Annoyed, drivers made unkind gestures.

"Asshole!" followed a long horn honk as one aggravated motorist passed.

"Get outta the street," another yelled, frustrated by the delay we caused.

Others shouted mean comments. Residents ignored volunteers distributing informational flyers explaining our Ride to Washington and ALS. Donations in this wealthy community were as rare as snowballs in the Sahara.

Later, everyone shared observations about the negative reception received in town. This was our first experience in populated areas outside the Metropolitan area. With so much cynicism and insanity in the world, nothing should surprise us. However, we did not expect it here. Over a roadside lunch made by supporters from central Jersey and a bathroom break at the Battle of Princeton National Monument commemorating Washington's defeat of the British, each told example after example of selfish behavior displayed by people in this community.

It was obvious; many residents did not want us in their town. Their concerns were what mattered to them at the moment. They cared little about the disease or the legitimate urgency of the cause. We pissed them off by delaying traffic for ten minutes or forcing them to move over a step in the sidewalk. It was that simple. If it did not involve them, they did not care. How sad. What is momentary inconvenience compared with an incurable, terminal illness?

I wanted to ask, "Like to trade places?"

After lunch, we started the last leg of day two which started in Elizabeth, New Jersey, about thirty miles away. By car, it was a short drive from Princeton to Trenton 15 miles down the road. It took us over two hours by wheelchair. Our coordinator called ahead to contact the police. They met us on the outskirts of the city. I reviewed the route and they questioned the decision to go straight through the city. They pointed out the area was poor, blighted and riddled with crime. In their opinion, it was not safe. They recommended a longer route bringing us to the Capital Building and skirting the inner city neighborhoods,

"Really?" I replied. Time was short and our plan was the most direct route to State House. "I want to go the shortest route."

Charlie said to them, "If we got through New York City okay, we will be good going through Trenton."

With their reluctant approval, we pressed onward through the city as planned. The once - bustling city appeared a ghost town. Row upon row of buildings were empty. I saw entire blocks razed, burned or boarded up. Pockets of people popped up.

We must have been an odd sight. Two wheelchairs riding down the center of the street, a couple of bicyclists, followed by a motor home all flanked by police surely stood out. Street corners were crowded with people milling. Curious kids were everywhere. As we pushed further, the more notice we attracted. We became an interesting spectacle. Folks came to their front doors to investigate the slow moving commotion.

"What is this?" residents asked. They wanted to know who I was and what I was doing.

I shouted, "I am traveling to Washington. I have Lou Gehrig's disease." My explanation moved the questioners.

"You have got to be kidding," said one Trentonian. "Man, that's awesome!"

We began getting hi-fives, head nods, and broad smiles of encouragement. Dollar bills waved in the air. The poorest were the most generous.

Of course, not everyone cared. Some ignored us. We heard a nasty comment occasionally, including a racist slur. I assumed some long-suffering people resented our intrusion with the police escorts when most of the time their community is neglected. We saw drug dealers. It was not a pretty sight. Nonetheless, the vast majority were welcoming, curious and supportive.

"Riding through the ghetto was the right decision. It was the best choice after all," I remarked to the team.

At the evening's planning session, the conversation centered on the stark contrasts of the day. The differences were startling, ironic and sobering. Everyone on the Ride had the same general opinions and conclusions.

"They can keep their town," a volunteer said referring to Princeton.

Those most capable of effecting change in research—the affluent—gave us the worst reception. In Princeton, we intruded in their lives with an agenda they were too busy to hear. Their world taught them to be cynical and unfazed. Blinded by myopic vision, they had little interest in us. Indifference and intolerance replaced the support we sought.

The residents of the inner city had little and few resources. Signs of poverty were everywhere. Their suffering was palpable. Despite their circumstance, or maybe because of it, they opened hearts and wallet. They embraced our suffering. Although separated by experience and culture from the minorities in Trenton, we felt more accepted and welcomed than in Princeton.

The Bible says, "We know that suffering produces perseverance; perseverance, character; and character, hope."

Suffering crushes some. Others never suffered. In either case, they lose or never develop one of the most powerful human characteristics. They have no hope.

The ALS Ride for Life is about hope.

The lesson I learned from this was not to assume wealth and power, i.e., the shakers and movers of society, will easily welcome new agendas outside their comfort zone. Those with the least may be the most receptive.

Jeannette of 2900 North

When economists and planners use the term "Rust Bucket" to describe the Northeast they chose well. At one time three generations ago, cities of the Northeast were thriving business bastions of the American economy. Time left them behind for lands to the south, southwest and west coast.

Philadelphia was once the third largest city in the nation and Baltimore was sixth. Between New York and Washington was one enormous powerhouse of industrial strength. It was a never-ending strip of industrial development. Smokestacks belched, refineries flowed, and trains rolled. Factories hummed and Americans worked.

In geographic area, Philadelphia remains a large city. It's boundaries blend with smaller adjoining cities, creating a continuous sprawl. Industries used to ring the outskirts of each city. As we rode through the region, the reason for the name "Rust Bucket" became glaringly apparent. It was a repeat of our initial experience in Trenton, except this area was on steroids.

"Man, I can't believe what I am seeing," I said to the volunteer biking with me. The sights rolling by us shocked me.

Numerous hulks of dead factories littered the entire way. Major population decline emptied the residential areas. Surviving neighborhoods were reduced to scattered buildings surrounded by vacant weed choked lots. An occupied home stood alongside boarded up or burned out shells. Abandoned cars decayed in open fields. Being there, I did not feel it was 1998.

"This seems like I am looking back at war torn Europe." I commented.

"Or a futuristic scene from an apocalyptic movie," he countered. "A big contrast to our upper class communities back home for sure."

South of Philly, we went through the city of Chester. Poverty was evident everywhere I rode. To us, it appeared another city struggling to survive. It was a visceral experience riding in the community. It rained non-stop so we dressed in our brilliant yellow rain gear at the hotel before we left. We prepared for these contingencies. A major outdoor clothing company, Helly Hansen donated 16 sets of foul weather gear. The day never brightened, setting a suitable mood as I rolled over the streets. I saw a broken city, filled with broken people crushed by the weight of poverty.

Even in the dreary weather, life managed to continue for the residents. Young men gathered in front of candy stores. Everywhere people walked or rode bicycles. Small groups collected on porches. My caravan attracted much attention, prompting curious stares. I smiled, waved and explained I was dying from Lou Gehrig's disease.

I shouted, "I'm on my way to Washington!" generating many good wishes.

The bystanders became engaged and encouraging. By mid-afternoon, the rain grew heavy, pelting my face. I experimented with attaching an umbrella to the chair but the winds

and people's need to talk with me made the umbrella imprac-
tical. I was on a mission so I asked someone to pull my hood
straps tight to keep out the driving rain. I endured the nasty
weather as I do my ALS. It scattered most of the residents.

I buried my exposed skin under my hood and tilted my
head downward to shelter from the stinging drops. I rolled
forward into the rain close behind my police escort. Because
of my hood, I could not see more than ten yards ahead. The
darkening street gleamed under the wet coat of rain. The
flashing red and blue emergency lights reflected off the shiny
pavement. I stared blindly into the hypnotic image and rode
on. The solitude soothed my soul.

An officer startled me by stepping up on my side.
"Someone wants to talk with you up the block. Is that okay?"
he asked.

Taken back by the surprising request I answered, "Sure!"

"Ok, when we get near, I'll pull the group over and you
can talk," he explained.

I pulled my hood back to look forward. Ahead, a knot of
people gathered at the curb. When I was across from them,
the police officer came back and motioned me over. He halted
the rest of the caravan. I smiled at the group and pointed my
chair towards them.

"Hello," I greeted them. A man in his mid-thirties came
forward.

"My mother wanted to talk to you," he told me. He
turned, took a few steps down the sidewalk and hopped up
the stoop disappearing through the door. A few minutes later,
a woman emerged from the house. She shuffled toward my
chair. I noticed her cropped, snow-white hair. She moved

with a slight hunch. Her steps were slow and deliberate. I waited a minute for her to cover the short distance from the stoop to the curb.

Her son introduced his mother, "My mom, Jeannette."

She smiled and greeted me with, "Hello, my son saw you passing by the stores back there and hurried home on his bicycle to tell me. He knew I would want to see you. God bless you for what you are doing," she said thrusting an envelope into my hand.

"I am happy to meet you," I replied.

"I want you to have this. It is all I can afford but I want to help you."

I moved to look into her eyes. "Thank you, Jeannette. My name is Chris. I am going to die from Lou Gehrig's disease. I am riding to end this nightmare," I explained.

She seemed to relate to me. "God bless you, Jeannette. We both have our journeys. Good luck to you on yours. May I please have a hug?"

She leaned and I stood because at that time my legs were still strong. We embraced one another, longer than a routine hug. I felt her light squeeze and I pressed in return. My fingers pushed into her frail frame. We were a sight I am sure, two strange souls embracing in the rain.

Anxious to move the procession along, the police approached. Following the cue, I turned to resume my Ride. I choked on my goodbye to Jeanette.

The sidewalk crowd evaporated as I steered back into the street. I did not look back; it was too painful. The rain poured. I buried my face once again and headed south. I clutched the envelope with cold, soaked fingers.

As I rolled in the rain, I thought about her and me. We bonded as strangers. On the outside, we were different in every respect. She was in her twilight while I was in the prime of life. She was infirmed and I, in relative health at that point. She was poor: I solid middle class. She lived in a deplorable house: I lived in a comfortable home. We were urban vs. suburban. She was a woman. I am a man. She was African American. I was Caucasian. She had to struggle against racism. I grew up privileged. Yet, for all that separated us, some things more powerful and universal united us.

We both refused to allow circumstance to dictate our life. We refused to give up. We looked to the future with optimism for tomorrow. We chose to be agents of change. We were kind, supportive and accepting of one another.

The most important was we each held on to hope.

I never opened Jeannette's envelope. The amount of its contents was not important. What it represented was far more significant than the money. I retold Jeannette's story many times. I wish her son could read this tribute to his mother. Over the years and in the turbulence of living with ALS, I have misplaced her envelope.

Perhaps that was for the best. Temptation may have caused me to open it. Not knowing its contents was a gift. Freed from reality, my imagination could soar conjuring contents beyond measure. Her envelope contained whatever we wanted it to be.

Jeannette reminded me of a fundamental truth. Hope is priceless. Thanks for the refresher, Jeannette.

The lesson I learned from this was hope transcends all circumstances in life. It is the power that drives grit and perseverance. It underpins the will and struggle to survive.

My Wife's Recipe

Even though you wanted oranges, life may give you lemons. When you are unable to make sweet orange juice, make lemonade and sweeten it with sugar.

With the congested urban centers of the Northeast behind, we had the peaceful rural farm stretches of Delaware and Maryland's eastern shore ahead. We pressed towards Dover, the second capital city of three we planned to visit. Two days away from the city, my wife received a phone call from its Chief of Police.

"You cannot go through the City as planned," the spokesperson said. "If you still want to come through Dover, you must give us an alternate route and avoid the Eastside of town."

"That stinks," she thought, we had so little time to create a reroute. "Why was that necessary?" Christine asked.

"Ma'am, the President is coming to speak at Dover Air Force Base and the City will be on lock down." Her wheels spun. Before she hung up, she was already making lemonade! She called us on the road.

I took her call while riding in northern Delaware, "Hello."

She was coy, saying, "I have bad news and good news."

Taking the bait, "Yeah, what do you have?" I said.

"The bad news is Bill Clinton is coming to Dover. The police need a new route avoiding the Eastside of the City, ASAP.

I shouted, "Shit! That stinks. So, gimme the good news."

"The good news is Bill Clinton is coming to Dover!"

I was confused. "How the hell is that good?" I barked. All I thought of were the headaches we had now because of his appearance.

"Now you can meet the President! He is visiting Dover Air Force Base. We have to figure out a way to get you in the audience."

Bill Clinton was coming to the Air Force Base to receive the bodies of several US soldiers killed in the Middle East. The somber reception ceremony was by invitation. The audience was military personnel and family members. It did not seem she could get me an invitation.

Against the odds, she spent the next 36 hours trying. She started with a lead obtained from the ALS Association. Phone calls to various agencies in Washington punctuated her day. Then, she hit the mother lode when she connected with the Secret Service security handling the President's visit to Dover.

At home, the next day raced for her. On the road, I crawled toward the City. Thinking about meeting the President, I rocketed from euphoria to disappointment and back contemplating if this would happen. Behind the scenes, angels were at work.

A call from the White House was the first indication an invitation was possible.

"We need a complete list and address of everyone involved in the Ride," they told Christine. "Background checks will be scheduled for the entire team. Is that a problem, ma'am?" the voice inquired.

That evening, we screamed in the hotel as we heard her update. We were drunk with excitement.

I tossed all night. Could it be possible I will see the President? The reception was on Saturday. Will we have enough time? My answer came the next morning.

Late the following day, the White House made it official.

"Mrs. Pendergast, your party will be given two tickets to attend President Clinton's address at Dover Air Force Base," she was informed by the Secret Service.

"Chris, get out your good pants and shoes. You're going to meet the President," she told me.

This was a powerful chance for awareness. Wearing our Ride tee shirts, mingling with important people and spreading the story was a special opportunity. The dilemma I faced: whom should I take to use the other pass? There was Fernando, the PALS who accompanied me most of the last two weeks. He wanted to go and felt he earned the opportunity.

The father in me pulled me towards my son. He has been at my side for the whole Ride. His young legs biked, walked or roller-bladed all the way. He threw his heart and soul into the Ride. ALS stole me from him. He grew up forced to share me. The friend in me tugged for Charlie. He sacrificed two weeks of his life to go with me and handled all the logistical details to get us here.

"I feel like Solomon trying to choose among worthy choices," I confided to Christine, "no matter the selection, someone will be disappointed."

Christine and I talked forever on the phone about my choices. Her wisdom helped me realize the validity of choosing my son.

"Family is forever," she reminded me. "Our family made the Ride happen. We bore the burdens of your advocacy work over years." She helped me decide my son would accompany me. She heard my angst about Charlie, who toiled endless days to make the Ride work.

"Let's try to get Charlie into the audience through a 'backdoor' plan," she proposed. We hatched a scheme to get one additional person in.

She and I rehearsed our plan. My twelve-year-old son was not capable of handling an emergency. I needed a caregiver; the Presidential audience was no different. The two passes we received were for guests, not medical personnel. We planned to arrive with three people; two guests, a medical assistant and hope for the best. Brilliant if it worked!

"Let's give it a shot," I said. Fate was now in control.

Bill Papaleo, a friend from back home was spending his second weekend with us. He was an avid bicyclist and rode many miles at my side. On the first weekend our delay cost us our police escort once we crossed the GW Bridge. I pressed on alone through the teeming streets of New Jersey just west of Manhattan. It rained lightly making the night come earlier. Bill rode at my side and thank God he did. In the darkening light, I ran through what I thought was a simple puddle.

It turned out to be a deep, water-filled pothole. I remember seeing the stores' neon signs turning sideways. I tipped over because of the crater. I wound up sprawled in the wet streets in between buzzing cars. My chair pinned me. I laid there unable to get up. Dozens of good Samaritans surrounded me, all shouting in Spanish. They were calling 911 for an ambulance. They mistook my paralysis for a serious injury. Bill did his best to explain I was fine. To his credit, he was able to make them understand and the "bus" was cancelled. He got me up, back in my chair. Bruised and banged up a little, both of us continued into the night. He was back to help the second week.

"Bill, I need your help again!"

"What do ya need?" he asked.

"Can you help me get Christopher ready to meet the President?" I asked.

From first responder he became a fashion buyer. He set out on a mission to find suitable clothes for my son to replace his ripped jeans and ragged sneakers.

When we arrived on Saturday, tight security ringed the Base. Police roamed like marauding locust. Helicopters thumped over us. Armed military lined every access point. Angry looking dogs prowled, held in check by tissue thin leashes. I was not sure if I got reassured or worried by the sights.

Our van eased to the checkpoint at the entrance. They stopped us. We told them the whole story. They inspected the vehicle twice. Black eye-glassed men peered at our identification and into the van at us. Christopher had none but his name appeared on their list. After questioning him, heads nodded and gates opened.

"Follow the marked roads," they told us.

We steered towards an isolated area on the outer part of the Base.

"Will you look at the size of that building?" Charlie gasped.

A cavernous hanger housing B-52s appeared ahead. The audience assembled outside. Numerous lines and temporary tents were set up. The van drove to the designated handicapped parking section. The ramp lowered, I held my breath and rolled the chair onto the tarmac.

I began praying, "God, please let my son and good friend have this extraordinary experience."

We cued up outside the building with the others waiting to get in to see the President. Maybe my chair and neck brace might evoke some sympathy I thought. I hoped it generated a warm, encouraging smile. It did not have any effect.

"Passes," a stone cold voice demanded.

We stood looking at him. All around the crowd stirred with anticipation. The atmosphere was electric. However, we appeared as if we were about to be electrocuted!

Charlie handed him two. "Where is the third?" he demanded.

"Agent?" Charlie attempted to speak. His glare burned through Charlie's eyes shutting him down.

Even though I sat, my knees buckled. I tried to shift the focus to me.

I chimed in, "Agent, there are only two of us, my son and me. The man with me is my medical assistant, not a guest. I cannot be left alone. I must travel with help," (which was true sort of).

Once I warmed up talking, I went into high gear and threw everything at him. I machine-gunned the entire Ride story in under a minute. He seemed to waiver.

Christopher pled his case too. "My father needs Charlie's help."

The line grew behind us as he deliberated. In unison, we all stared at the harried Secret Service Agent.

"Go ahead," he announced. Thank you Lord. And, thanks Christine!

We sat in the hanger along with the other guests and listened. President Clinton addressed the families of the deceased soldiers. It was emotional as the President embraced each family member after speaking. His team motioned to the security detail to bring the audience down from the bleachers and over to the ropes separating the President. He wanted to greet some of them as he departed. Hallelujah, another window opened.

The handicapped section, by some miracle, was right at the rope barrier! I was in perfect position to meet the President in person. Lemonade indeed!

Each greeter shook his hand and exchanged pleasantries. The encounters lasted at most, a few seconds. I doubt these guests had an agenda. We were on a mission. When the President approached, Charlie assisted me to stand up from my chair. Christopher was at my side.

The President extended his hand expecting another routine well-wisher. I seized the opportunity and clung to him like a stripe on a zebra. I brought up my other hand and clamped on him. I noticed half a dozen alarmed Agents hover closer.

The President went into his routine of pumping his arm. Like an old-fashioned water well, it drew my words up. As water from the pump, they flowed from my mouth: ALS, lack of medicine, absence of awareness, my diagnosis, my wheel-chair Ride to Washington, and my goal to find a cure. He nodded in approval as I explained. My words engaged him.

"Yes, I am familiar with ALS. I lost a good friend," the President said.

I brought Christopher to his attention. My son was standing next to me decked out in his new threads. I relived how he traveled the whole way at my side on foot, bike and skates. I released my grip. The President turned to him.

"You are quite a brave young man. Congratulations," he said as he shook Christopher's hand. They bantered a bit.

"Mr. President, may we show you our tee shirt?" He smiled, as I opened up a tee. He held it to examine it as I detailed the stops along the fourteen-day journey. I asked him, "Will you please wear it?" He smiled again.

It took me several minutes to wrap up. Mission accomplished! Awareness achieved.

A reporter came to me and remarked, "You spoke a long time to the President. What did you say?"

I repeated most of what I said. We left for Annapolis the next day. I never found what, if anything, the reporter did with the interview. I hope he passed it on in a story for readers in Dover.

Once we returned home, Charlie developed the beautiful photos he took documenting the day. We selected three of our favorites and framed them. The first was the President and I. The second, Christopher and Clinton. The final, the President examining our shirt.

In our non-ALS world, my wife was a veteran labor advocate in her local teacher union. She had the distinction of being the first woman elected president of her local union, an affiliate of the New York State United Teachers. In this position, she developed useful connections. She attended meetings everywhere.

To court the labor vote, President Clinton planned to deliver the keynote address at the American Federation of Teachers National Convention coming during the summer. My wife sprung to action again.

She asked a senior-level union official to assist in getting her to meet the President at the New Orleans convention. She flew off to New Orleans on a mission: to get the pictures from the Ride signed.

She found out that after he spoke, President Clinton planned to "work the ropes." The day of the keynote address, she went two hours ahead of time to ensure a spot near the front of the auditorium. In her haste to be there in plenty of time, she forgot the photos in her room. By the time she realized, it was too late to leave because she would lose her spot.

In a Groundhog Day-like moment, Christine also wound up on the Presidential receiving line. When he came to her, she grabbed his hand. Her other hand also wrapped around him like a hungry octopus gripping a meal.

"Mr. President, you met my husband in Dover. He has ALS and rode his wheelchair to Washington," she said. His eyebrows rose and he slowed. She relayed more details.

Clinton's eyes caught hers. "Yes, I am aware of ALS. I lost a friend. It's a terrible disease. It sounds wonderful what he is doing."

He leaned forward and embraced her. With emphasis he added, "You stay strong." He broke off by saying, "I wish you my best." He moved down along the line interacting with the well-wishers. Christine floated for a few moments absorbing the experience.

A bit down the line, President Clinton stopped and turned. He walked back up the line to Christine. The President reconnected with her. His sparkling blue eyes locked onto hers.

"I do remember your husband. Your boy was with him, right?" Her heart pounding with joy as he spoke.

She cried out, "Yes!"

The President met thousands of people in the months between the Dover meeting and the Union convention. How he remembered our son and the Dover meeting is beyond remarkable, she thought.

With a broad smile he added, "You tell that boy, he is a very special young man!"

It was an out-of-body experience for her.

The New York delegation was ecstatic when it heard the news of the meeting. The Ride was popular among educators in the Metropolitan area. She gave the photos to a union official who had connections with the White House. They would try to have them signed.

My wife returned home. She was thrilled to talk with the President, but frustrated that her mission went unfulfilled. Both of us were grateful for the privilege to meet and talk with our Nation's leader. We forgot about the photos. We had the memory. We resumed our lives.

Months later, a registered mail notice arrived. She went to sign and pick up the mail. It was from the White House. Inside were her photos. President Clinton signed them. He personalized each. They hang on our wall reminding us to make lemonade when we get lemons.

On that day, what a delicious lemonade she made.

Nowadays, I have a feeding tube. When I first got it in 2013, I was losing weight and had GI problems. Tube feedings sustained me for a year until I recovered enough to resume eating by mouth. However, I continue to use the tube for hydration. Drinking fluids in large volumes is quite difficult for me. I sip iced tea in the summer, hot tea in the winter and of course, an occasional glass of Guinness any time. On the rarest of occasions, I get to savor lemonade.

The tube needs to be changed. A small balloon about one-half the size of a golf ball anchors my type of device into my stomach. Over time, the powerful stomach acids eat away at the latex causing the balloon to leak. Once by accident a caregiver pulled it out.

I used to go to the ER and wait endless hours for someone to insert a temporary catheter line. Then later I went to a GI doctor for an actual feeding tube replacement. My brave and strong wife learned how to do a tube replacement at home. My replacement procedure is now quick and convenient. She gets the bonus of being able to inflict a small amount of pain on me to make up for all my annoying behaviors.

She then quips, "That will be $4,000 please."

"You will have to take it out in trade." I reply. Boy, what a life we have!

I tell a fictional black humor story of when the doctor told me I needed a feeding tube put in and I would have to stop eating by mouth.

"Thank God," I exclaimed.

The astonished doctor said, "Well, that's a first! I never had that reaction before."

I smiled, "Doctor, you would shout 'Thank God' too, if you had to eat my wife's cooking!"

The truth be told, not only does my wife make delicious lemonade, her cooking is excellent. I love all of my wife's recipes.

The lesson I learned from this was adversity is not necessarily an impediment to success. It can be an opportunity to achieve greater results. It epitomizes the expression, make lemonade when you get lemons.

Treasures

The stretch on Maryland's Eastern Shore sandwiched between Dover and the Chesapeake Bay is an isolated agricultural area. Small roads wind through the spring's chest-high corn, oats and hay fields. The huge fields hid quaint, tiny towns. The deeply grooved shoulder of the road contained mysterious long, narrow, parallel ruts.

"Man, these are a pain in the neck. I can't keep my damn chair straight," I bellyached.

The ruts made my wheels drift in and out, making an uncomfortable ride. The peculiar grooves clarified as I passed the first pile of manure. Then, on the horizon appeared a black silhouetted box. In no time, the distinct shape of a horse formed. It was a buggy. The bearded driver sped by, steering the horse drawn carriage off the shoulder into the road when he passed me.

"Ah, mystery solved." I said. "We are in Amish country."

What an unusual juxtaposing occurrence. An 18th century horse carriage passing a 20th century state of the art medical scooter. Next, a wagon drove by filled with a large family. The curious children studied me with inquisitive eyes. I smiled and nodded to acknowledge their interest. The stoic adults looked forward, avoiding eye contact.

The Ride entered a bustling Amish community. Amish farmhouses situated in lush fields lined both sides for a solid hour. Their homes were unusual because there were no wires or electric poles leading to them from the road. I wondered the fate and life of an ALS patient in their community.

The tracks faded and manure piles grew infrequent, then stopping all together. Modern farmers atop mechanized equipment replaced the idyllic sight of a score of people working on fertile fields each using some interesting but bygone hand tool.

Because we were traveling through on a weekend, a large contingent of family and friends from home joined us. The Maryland State Troopers, wheelchairs, escorting bicyclist, Christopher on roller blades, my handicapped van bedecked with slogans and a motor home along with several cars, all combined to make quite an impression on the sleepy farm communities.

Traffic slowed to a snail's pace as we passed. Eye bulging drivers attempted to read the signs on the motor home or the white washed letters scrawled on my handicapped van. The escorting bicyclist or my son answered the questions of stopping motorists. I focused on covering the ambitious mileage goal set for the day: 25.

"A woman just passed us," a volunteer told me.

"Yeah, and?" I replied waiting to hear the rest of the details.

"She is pulling off the road up ahead where there is more room," he continued.

"How come?"

"She said she was driving the other way, saw us and turned around. She wants to make a donation," the volunteer grinned.

When I heard the message, I became excited. I anticipated a contribution. Roadside donations pumped everyone up and fueled us for the next section of road. I was eager to meet her. As she promised, she pulled off the road to await me. Her persistence impressed me, elevating my expectations.

I wheeled over to her old, beat up car. She was mid-thirties and not well dressed. She opened the door to speak.

"I was impressed with what you are doing," she said. Going on she told me, "I do not know anyone with it, but I wanted to help you find a cure."

Stepping out and slipping her hand into her jeans, she pulled out a pocket full of change. Her hand balled around the coins and she extended the fistful to me.

"I have even more!" Hurriedly, she bent down and returned to the car. I watched her lean over the console, tearing it up searching for other loose change. She gathered a few more coins. Exiting with a smile typical of a kid finding a hidden treasure, she surrendered her booty.

"Thank you," I told her as I accepted her offering. "That is very generous and kind. This will help."

Satisfied, the woman got in her car and drove away. I returned to the road. Driving through the peaceful farm country undistracted by whizzing automobiles, red lights or the stop and go traffic found in towns, I covered many miles. I thought about our roadside donors. What motivated them?

By outward measurements, this woman was not a person of means. There was no connection to ALS. Yet, she gave everything she had, scraping the bottom. Not embarrassed by her modest contribution, she chose to share and make a difference. It epitomizes the best charitable spirit. She gave as the Bible instructs, not from abundance, rather from scarcity. How genuine and authentic.

I tossed the pile of change in my pocket. At day's end, we pooled all the donations. Nobody counted her donation separately. That was not necessary. The amount did not matter. Her gift was enormous in symbolism. We spoke of the incident many times since. It became something of a legend from the beginning days.

We labeled it our gold standard of selfless giving. If people would give in similar spirit, the world of ALS would be a much brighter place. A cure would be found much sooner.

The lesson I learned from this was the value of something can exceed its obvious monetary amount. Even small contributions are meaningful. Any amount becomes significant. Give whatever you can with joy.

Oh Say Can You See

Baltimore has played an important role in American history. It gave us our national anthem. It's also important in the formation of The ALS Ride for Life organization.

Planning for the first Ride, I struggled to get responses from various organizations. I was an unknown entity, championing an unknown cause. How would I get increased awareness and more pragmatically, how would I gather support and volunteers? How would I get wheelchair manufacturers to loan equipment and persuade hotels to donate rooms, for example? I was frustrated but not discouraged. I aimed high and continued.

"I need some name recognition associated with us," I shared with my team.

I thought a premier ALS research institution would impart some credibility to our event. I wrote Dr. Rothstein a young, eager physician with a growing reputation as a researcher at Johns Hopkins University Hospital in Baltimore, and explained my plan. He came to Hopkins as a resident in neurology in 1986, became a faculty member three years later and opened his own lab at the hospital. I requested a reception and tour of the lab.

"Dr. Rothstein, we would like to stop by the lab and perhaps see some of your work," I told him in an email.

He responded right away. "We would love to have you visit."

When we reached Baltimore on the second week of the Ride in 1998, we moved north through downtown and towards Hopkins. The previous day we had been in the third capital of the trip, Annapolis, which is south of the city. Dr. Rothstein greeted us with a huge smile and open arms. Another patient, Fernando was with me.

Aware of our tiny size, "We are small in number but mighty in spirit," I told the doctor.

"Welcome," he exclaimed walking over to our wheelchairs. His small frame squared the massive hospital behind him. He smiled and extended his arm to shake our hands. "Come inside, we are happy you are here." He continued, "This is wonderful what you are doing for the ALS community."

He was a gracious, affable man. He took his time showing us around his lab and talked about his research with excitement. Because I was inexperienced in the world of research and grant funding, I peppered him with endless questions. I wanted to know everything! With utmost patience, he answered every one.

I found out that grants fall far short of keeping a lab up and running. Many mundane but important items are outside grant funds. These items are the nuts and bolts binding a lab team together—coffee, computer ink, postage, stationery and various supplies. I listened to his passionate words as I made mental notes. We enjoyed a nice lunch, took advantage of bathrooms and filled up on water before pressing on.

The doctor walked us to the street. "Good luck, Chris."

"Thanks, Doctor," I said, although my words were almost empty of significance when compared to the value the stop had for me. We were off. Washington, the end of our journey, was a scant 40 miles south.

I was so impressed with Dr. Rothstein. I vowed to help him somehow. When the Ride was over and we returned home, I set out to fulfill my promise. Without trying, my awareness Ride managed to raise money. This came as a surprise to everyone. I directed the money we raised go to the ALS Association of Greater New York. They were the only group willing to help me and committed their funds to get me to Washington. Their boldness and empowerment of patients turned out far better than imagined. For their support, we earned $30,000 for them. I saw this as my opportunity to help Dr. Rothstein.

"I want to send Dr. Rothstein some money for his lab." I told the president of the chapter. Little did I expect the reaction to my request. I wanted 10% of the $30,000 be sent to Hopkins.

"We can't do that," the president informed me. "Dr. Rothstein will have to apply for a grant like everyone else."

In protest I said, "I raised the money, can't I help determine how it is spent?" I was flabbergasted.

"We have to follow our regulations to receive a grant," she said. "I am sorry."

We never discussed what to do with any money we raised prior to the event because it was unexpected that we would come out ahead. We both assumed the Ride event would run on a deficit requiring their funding. I was grateful for the pledge of support. Without it, it's doubtful the Ride as we know it would exist. I was torn and frustrated.

"We are bound by the guidelines of the organization. We cannot make an exception for you. I'm sorry." The president was sympathetic but unmoving.

They did not send the mini grant. I did not argue or become belligerent. I thought of the old proverb, "Fool me once, shame on you. Fool me twice, shame on me." I decided, if I ever did this or something similar, I would never relinquish control of the income I sweated and worked so hard to raise. I needed my own organization giving me control of our donations. A fundamental foundation of that organization would be to empower patients who were helping to raise money to have a voice in how it is spent.

Similar to how Christine reacted to my initial plan to do the first Ride, my wife prohibited me from using the 'N' word around her. However, it was almost impossible not to say. Try as I might, it slipped out often. Everyone expected the Ride not to go beyond one year. They assumed my strength would deteriorate fast like normal. They should have thought again!

In my head, I planned for the *next* one soon after returning home. I was committed for life, as long as that would be. However, the next time, I would be the master of my own fate. I might not have control over what was happening to my body, but I was determined to have control of things I did.

On the second trip to Baltimore, we visited Hopkins again and this time we could commit to donating money. For the 1999 Ride to Washington, I formed an independent organization to manage everything. I was able to give Dr. Rothstein a modest $2,500.

In 2000, Dr. Rothstein opened the Packard Center for ALS Research, destined to become a leading international consortium of ALS researchers. The hallmark of the Center was its collaborative approach. He required sharing of research as part of the grant process for recipients. He set the stage for the future of ALS research: Teamwork and collaboration. In total, the ALS Ride has donated almost a half million dollars to Dr. Rothstein's Packard Center for their research.

By opening up to us, Dr. Rothstein did more than he realized. His affirming welcome greased the skids to propel us further than either dreamed. Thanks, Doctor.

In addition to Hopkins, we also made a home plate appearance at a Baltimore Orioles baseball game. While at the stadium, a small number of PALS met us. Among them was Larry Katz, a prominent lawyer in Washington. We talked about my experience with rigid national groups and my organization. He offered to help.

"I'll help you incorporate pro bono, Chris," Larry said.

What a gift! By the end of the year, The Ride for Life was official. Three years later, thanks to Larry's hard work, we received tax-exempt status from the IRS. Since then, we have received an amazing amount of more than $8,500,000 in direct donations and another $1,000,000 given to other organizations on our behalf.

When we formulated the by-laws for incorporation, it specified approximately 50% of our budget be for research, 40% earmarked for patient services and 10% devoted to raising awareness or education. This split was a compromise brought about by others helping me plan and execute the

Ride. We named our nursing assistance program, 'Katz Care' in his honor. Larry died shortly after accomplishing his goal.

As promised, others were encouraged to voice suggestions. If they raise money, they help spend it. Most notable, PALS help direct the research funds.

As a more robust patient, I focused on finding a treatment or cure. I did not experience the agonizing struggles patients endure every day. Growing up watching John Wayne's war and western movies, I had the mentality of, "I am already mortally wounded, don't waste anything on me, I'm not gonna make it."

In my mind, resources should go to those who have a chance: Future patients not yet diagnosed. I favored spending everything on research to end this scourge. Originally, I intended to spend nothing on services. Research would get all the money we raised.

Nancy Venditti along with her brother Bob Cauttero lobbied hard to spend money for patient care. Not long ago, the pair lived the hardship inflicted by the cruel progression of ALS. It was raw and fresh in their minds. They wanted to continue working on the mission and I needed the help. Both were valuable getting the Ride on the road. I acquiesced recognizing their contributions. The split budget allocation was established. That compromise changed the course of the Ride's future.

That groundbreaking decision enabled a variety of patient services such as the establishment and annual funding of Long Island's single ALS Clinic, a wonderful development providing needed services. Created as a partnership between ALS Association of Greater New York and State University of

New York at Stony Brook, it opened in 2002. We fund the clinic by providing money to pay for the Nurse Coordinator. Theresa Imperato is the pivotal person making the clinic run well and helping patients navigate the bewildering world of ALS.

"Theresa is the glue holding the clinic together," I once remarked when describing the clinic operation. "Without her, patients would be lost."

The clinic has grown from operating one day a month with one physician in the beginning, to running one day a week with three doctors today. Since the inception, our organization has donated close to $900,000 to underwrite its operations.

Several years after the clinic was established, it was renamed, The Christopher K. Pendergast ALS Center of Excellence. Our Honorary Chairman David Cone, retired Yankee pitcher, presided over the naming ceremony to the delight of 325 attendees.

"As honorary chairperson of ALS Ride for Life, it gives me great pleasure to announce the official name of the clinic at Stony Brook University Hospital is now the Christopher K. Pendergast Center of Excellence." David announced to the crowd.

The experience overwhelmed me. I filled with joy and wonderment at how this all came to be. It is a strange feeling to go to the clinic for my visit and see the brass plaque with my name on it. After the moment's pride, I think of all the lives of Ride participants who have fallen, 85 men and women since I began the journeys. I recall all the volunteers who worked so hard to keep the organization alive. I remember all the generous businesses.

The most important remembrance, my wife Christine, who has been at my side through it all. It seems unfair that just my name is on the plaque.

Due in large part to Nancy and Bob, over 1,000 patients have received vital support from ALS Ride For Life, through our patient service programs. We provide nursing grants across the nation, as well as legal assistance grants for insurance and end-of-life issues. In our region, we have a fleet of handicapped vans for short/long-term loan, mobility devices, scholarships for students affected through a family member with ALS, and a caregiver support group. Our social worker delivers these services with skillful guidance.

I told Nancy and Bob, "Your father is proud of his two kids. So am I."

Like our anthem, it started in Baltimore. Long may Baltimore wave.

The lesson I learned from this was physicians dispense more than medicine to promote health. Sometimes it is how they act and what they do that also have a positive impact on a patient's outcome.

In My Daughter's Eyes

On the first few Rides to Washington, I had another very important helper. In fact, the helper has been involved with ALS since birth and has a special place in my heart. This helper's story began May 5, 1977 with the birth of our daughter, sweet Melissa.

The smooth swaying in shaded summer air worked every time. Nestled between my chest and soft ample belly, she dozed securely, reassured by my heart beating a familiar pulse. A screaming infant and an exasperated new father transformed into a serene pair of hammock bound bums. Ah, the memories. I can't pass a hammock and not remember.

Mother Nature was my go-to person for soothing my troubled spirit. It made sense to bring my daughter to her as well. My wife and I took our daughter everywhere outdoors. Melissa rode in my backpack up to the summit of Blue Mountain, in the Adirondack Mountains of New York her first summer. Tucked in the fabric safe and secure, she stared cooing periodic approval.

She survived a harrowing intrusion by a foraging black bear. It awoke us one summer night as we camped at the base of the mountain. The three of us slept in our tent. Melissa was bundled in her playpen with Christine and me snuggling in our sleeping bag.

"Honey, wake up!" she whispered.

A violent windstorm shook us to consciousness. The walls of the tent trembled, threatening to collapse. I struggled to clear sleep's cobwebs and figure out why the frame heaved up and down.

"Snort."

I had my answer. It came again in another loud, clear, unmistakable sound.

"Snort," a creature grunted.

My heart accelerated from rest to cardiac arrest territory in a flash. The snorting followed with sounds of breaking glass. My terrified wife peered into the blackness.

I put my lips to her ear, "It's a bear!" I breathed.

We violated the cardinal rule of camping in bear country: NEVER leave food around your campsite. Now we were paying for forgetfulness. The bear clawed its way into the screened portion of the tent for the remains of last night's dinner, all wrapped and waiting.

"He's eating the leftovers," I said furious at our campmates who left the trash.

The storm I thought shaking the tent was the bear's thick, sharp, three and a half inch claws tearing though the nylon screening. Each new swat re-shook the flimsy tent.

The breaking sound was the lantern knocked to the ground by the hungry bear on the prowl for a midnight snack. What would he do after trashing our kitchen area? Would he enter the sleeping area next? We prayed the ruckus did not wake Melissa. All the bear needed to invite himself in was her cry.

The darkness compounded the terror. How can I protect my sleeping baby? We remained fixed by fear. I laid back imagining how to improvise a defense against an agitated 400-pound bear. The one weapon I could MacGyver was the aluminum legs of the camp cots. Not very formidable against the brute power of his bite.

"What should we do?" she wanted to know.

"Nothing, wait and pray!"

The tent rocked again on its exit. Wire–bristled fur scraped the thin canvas walls, signaling the bear circling us outside the tent. Its claws clicked against hard packed soil as it paced back and forth. We prayed and waited. Sometime later, I drifted off. Melly slept through the entire episode.

When she was a baby, I often walked holding her in my arms. I always pointed out the birds flying overhead.

"Hey Melissa, can you see the birds?" I asked her day after day. Next spring, she said her first word. It wasn't the customary Momma or Dadda.

One unexpected moment she uttered, "Bird!"

Her birth was unplanned. My school district awarded me a six-month sabbatical leave at full pay to study and develop environmental programs. I chose to expand it to an entire year at half pay. I was with my infant daughter as much as my wife. Melissa and I formed a close bond.

One day, Christine and I were sitting on the stoop watching our daughter play in the driveway. She tumbled and fell scraping her knee. The trickle of blood dripping from the cut terrorized her. She screamed bloody murder as she ran back toward us.

Wailing, she called, "Mommy, Mommy!" She followed with, "Daddy, Daddy!" Then, "Daddy, Mommy, Mommy, Daddy!" Her instinct to include me as a primary source of comfort deeply touched me.

We continued looking skyward. On summer evenings, I would point out Mars.

I would ask her, "Hey Melissa, can you see Mars?"

When she was ten, Halley's Comet returned to earth to a great fanfare. I dragged her up before dawn and headed to the beach to view the comet. We looked through some telescopes set up to view the rare visitor.

"Is that it?" she asked in an innocent voice of a tired ten-year-old.

Unimpressed at the distant blur, she crawled up on the floor of the car and fell asleep. I thought, so much for this history-making astronomy!

She befriended animals that I brought home from my nature center at school. To introduce her to a ferret, I had a plan.

"Put a dab of peanut butter on your index finger," I told her. Trusting my judgement, she did it.

"I will hold the ferret," I explained and brought it close.

Worried, she said, "Are you sure?"

"Yeah, it's fine, do it!"

She extended the covered finger. The animal licked the treat and liked it. He decided to take a nibble.

"Ooooww," she screamed and pulled her hand back scaring it.

Now frightened, he clamped down on her finger and held on. She swung her arm in the air with the ferret dangling below. Before I could pry his mouth open and release the finger, I had to stop her from flailing about. The more she continued, the harder it bit. She waved it around like a stage prop. After much begging (who'd trust me further?), she held still.

"I will pry open the mouth and he will let go," I told her. When I did, she grabbed her finger.

"That hurt," she said looking at two tiny puncture wounds. Ferrets are notorious nippers. She panicked and that frightened the animal who in turn frightened her. The curious nip turned into a real bite. I forced myself not to laugh at the calamity.

Melissa walked pigs, chased goats, gathered chickens, held rats, fed iguanas, and talked to parrots, all to assist me. I loved her childhood. She was a joy. During her mid-teens, the father she knew and loved had to leave her forever. ALS took that part of me from her. Nevertheless, a loving piece of me remained. She had no choice except share her new Dad with ALS. She gave up so much.

For example, the annual Ride coincides with her birthday every year. For 5 years, there were no big parties because we were on the road. I bought her first legal drink in some dumpy neighborhood bar in Baltimore.

"Happy Birthday, Melissa," I toasted her. We raised our bottles of beer and drank. I tried hard to make her life normal.

We shared the dream of walking down the aisle on her wedding day. By the time it came, I was no longer walking. I vowed not to deny her the dream. Practice makes perfect, so we rehearsed walking with assistance.

I arranged to sit in the third pew, close to the altar. Her Godfather, Tom Longo, escorted her up the aisle stopping at my pew. With two helpers, I rose and went to her. In reverse of tradition, my daughter held me up. Clutching my arm between both of hers, she walked me down the aisle. Dream accomplished, though not as we thought.

Nine months pregnant, my daughter still participated in the Ride 2007. On the first day, she sported with pride a homemade tee shirt.

"I'm walking for my grandpa," the tee shirt proclaimed.

She amazed everyone with her brisk strides day after day. The evening before the finishing day, my wife got a phone call.

"Mom, I'm having some cramps," she said.

"How far apart?" my wife asked.

"About every few minutes," she said. "I think I may have the baby next week."

My wife went wild, "Get to the hospital! You are already in labor."

I heard the words, get to the hospital. "What's going on?" I asked my wife.

"Get up, Melissa is having the baby," my wife shouted.

I never missed the last day of the Ride. I never had a grandchild either. We did not participate the last day but went straight to the hospital. Patrick was born in the wee hours Saturday morning. Melissa beamed.

With a broad grin, she told us, "My timing was perfect. You go back and finish the Ride!"

My wife called the Ride group who were eager to get a news update.

Elizabeth Hashagen announced to everyone, "It's a boy!"

Cheers broke out. With daughter and grandson doing well, we met up with everyone in the afternoon and finished the Ride.

Adversity is a double edge sword. True, ALS has taken a great deal it has also given much. Finding the positives in times of difficulty requires the faith and strength to look. For those who try, they discover a higher level of awareness. Life takes on new meaning. While the suffering remains, it's balanced by an acceptance leading to peace. Pleasure and joy exist alongside pain and loss. It is not unlike my favorite Chinese dish, Sweet and Sour Pork.

Prior to the birth, during the third trip to Washington in 2000, we organized a candlelit ecumenical memorial service at the Lincoln Memorial for fallen ALS patients. I calculated that the number of annual deaths divided by days and hours equaled about 90, which I began using as a sound bite. It went on our first stationery back in 1999. Ninety flames flickered around the front of the Tidal Pool at the base of Lincoln's imposing statue. The ninety signifies the number of minutes between ALS deaths.

I said, "I hope these people have not died in vain. Perhaps their sacrifice will hasten a cure."

At the end of the ceremony, my daughter held a burning candle and read a poem she wrote for me. Her words held spellbound the 150 gathered on this hallowed site. Her eyes teared and voice quivered.

"Sometimes I see my father, this man built tall and wide.
His family is his love, his life and his pride.
A man so brilliant, filled with wit and charm,

219

To no one would he ever do harm.

Sometimes I see my father, his eyes sparkling ever so blue,
but oh, how I know the pain of these stories so true
His heart once happy, always singing a song,
Just how did it happen, whatever went so wrong?

Sometimes I see my father, his summers spent pushing me on my
swing
Our entertainment? Well of course, we would sing!
At night we gazed up at the stars
As he exclaimed, "Hey toots, can you see Mars?"

From the beauty of every sunrise to every sunset....
From every creature and every mountain I would bet —
His impact on people no one will ever forget.

Sometimes I see my father, but always I see my hero."

I wept openly as I listened. Without this illness, my journey would have been quite different.

If men were honest, most would admit they want to be their little girl's hero. If women were honest, most would admit they want to be their daddy's princess.

How blessed I am. ALS helped make these wishes come true. She is my princess and I am a hero in my daughter's eyes.

The lesson I learned from this do your best to raise a child with love and respect. The rewards later are worth the effort. You produce a decent human being who will make you proud. That is a priceless feeling.

Stepping Up

After doing three trips to Washington and participating in National Advocacy Day on the Hill, it was time for a change. It was difficult to generate support in far off cities and the rural countryside. The Ride took tremendous effort; how could we maximize its impact?

We held a meeting with a health related public relations firm and they advised refocusing. They suggested we select a different venue. Rather than traveling where we could not provide preparatory or follow up activities, we decided to focus at the local level. The Ride would occur on Long Island.

"The Ride is switching routes," I announced. "We need to focus on our local communities. The 2001 Ride will take place in the Metro area."

The switch to the metro area brought major modifications. The most significant was it enabled the education community to become involved. It also gave an opportunity for new leadership to emerge.

In time, family and changing life demands drew Charlie in other directions. Another physical education teacher also from Dickinson, Kevin McGinn witnessed Charlie's work first hand. Curious, he too edged closer to the infamous "event horizon" and was sucked into the Ride's Black Hole.

When the Ride changed venues in 2001, he began helping on the Ride. A year later Charlie made his tough decision.

"I want to step down as coordinator of the Ride," he said to me. "It was a difficult decision. After four years, it is time." Kevin was ready to assume the mantle of leadership. He was young, driven, organized and as dedicated a man as Charlie. Whatever worry I had about his ability to step up to the level of excellence set by his predecessor evaporated on day one of his first solo Ride.

"Kevin, what a great first day," I confessed on day one of Ride 2002. "I had some doubts because Charlie was so good. But man, you got us to an excellent start."

He brushed off the compliment with, "Well, it's easy when you have a good team behind you." As most people associated with the Ride, he did not have a big ego. He shared the accolade with everyone.

He proved as solid and capable. Unlike Charlie, Kevin had two very young children. His wife taught math in one of our district's middle schools. Kevin's role became a family affair. All the McGinns joined. His son, Patrick, took over the "chair jockey" job when available. Kevin's wife, Donna made blankets with her church's religious education class. She gave the blankets to each PALS. They remain in use more than a dozen years after. I cherish mine and use it all the time. It is as bright and clear as the day she put the Ride logo on the blanket. She got her school to raise money.

Their youngest child, Maggie, grew up with the Ride and helped in many different ways. Maggie was a reliable road companion for many years. I recall an Italian Ice store named McGoo we passed and asking her if she owned it. I call her

Maggie McGoo ever since. Now a teacher herself, I wonder what her students would think if I came to her class and called her that name today.

Like Charlie, Kevin's life changed as his family grew up. New demands, coaching, and work responsibilities all conspired to draw him away from the Ride.

"Chris, I wrestled with this for a long time," he began.

I read his mind. I knew what was coming. "You want to stop running the Ride. I understand Kevin."

I didn't want to make it any tougher or more awkward than necessary. After a decade of devoted service, Kevin did more than his share. It was a blow but not a total surprise. Leadership is an isolating and thankless task. When you throw in no salary, it is a wonder anyone even does it at all. Still, there was disappointment mixed with concern.

I hoped the small, part time office staff, my wife and volunteers could fill the vacuum Kevin created. The Ride had a certain inertia, which would carry it forward for a time. Looking back on the decade Kevin led the Ride, it was an impressive run.

When we brought the Ride to Long Island in 2001, it had no credibility or influence. ALS remained little known to most and the Ride even less. Enlisting local support was a steep uphill battle. I turned to places where I already had some influence.

As a young boy, I loved history. I consumed everything I could on the subject. I followed government and politics.

"You should be a politician," I heard many times.

I followed Jacob Javits, New York's Republican Senator. I knew his courageous battle with this debilitating disease. Still able to walk but unable to breathe, he appeared connected to a ventilator for his Senate meetings. I watched his unsuccessful 1980 re-election bid. He ran as an independent because he lost the Republican nomination. Historians attribute the defeat in part due to Lou Gehrig's disease.

During the start of my career, I attended Stony Brook University on Long Island as a graduate student. I took many classes in the Javits Center. At that time, I never gave it a second thought. Now, 20 years later—as an ALS patient—my curiosity was piqued.

"Why did this building carry his name?" I asked but nobody seemed to know.

I researched Javits discovering he was instrumental in securing funding for Stony Brook University in its formative years. The University houses his Senate papers, office desk, rocking chair and flag in the library's Special Collections department. As an alum and ALS patient, I had a strong link with the University.

"Maybe they will be a logistical stop on the Ride?" I asked my planning team. "They have a strong incentive."

"I will help on that one," my friend Andy said. He was also an alum as well as an American History teacher in an area high school.

We contacted the University requesting they host a stop on the Ride. Janice Rohlf, vice president for governmental affairs returned the call.

A call came into the office. "May I speak to Mr. Pendergast please?" she said. At that time, the Ride office was located in our converted dining room. My assistant happened to be in working.

"One moment please," she answered, passing the phone to me.

"Hello, how can I help you?" I said.

"My name is Janice Rohlf. I am Vice president for governmental affairs at Stony Brook University. Dr. Shirley Kenny, the university president approved your request." We found out later Dr. Kenny was sympathetic because a member of her family had ALS.

Ray Manzoni, Andy MacAvoy and I met with Janice to begin planning. She became our contact person and we developed a strong connection. We made Stony Brook a stop on the inaugural LI Ride in 2001. The Javits Collection Room opened for PALS, families and volunteers to tour his memorabilia. It was emotional for me as I thought about the man behind the exhibit. Senator Javits set the bar high for PALS to follow. He demonstrated how to live and be productive with ALS. I try to follow his example.

Today Stony Brook University is a multi-level supporter and essential partner in the fight against ALS. This is a result of Janice. She opened herself and embraced our mission. She serves as our First Vice-Chair today, long after she retired from the University. Her legacy of caring and support on the campus continues now through President Dr. Samuel Stanley, Vice Presidents Dr. Kenneth Kaushansky (University Hospital) and Dexter Bailey (Stony Brook Foundation) as well as School of Social Welfare Dean Dr. Jacqueline Mondros. The ALS Clinic at University Hospital, our loaned office space, all the logistical assistance and the rigorous research at the University are all tributes to Janice's open heart and the current leadership at Stony Brook. Everything at SBU traces back to her efforts. She even enlisted her husband Jim. He was helpful developing and maintaining our computer and Web programs.

"Thank you, Janice." I have said often. "And thank you Stony Brook." I repeat it now.

Pre-college schools were also critical to the Ride's success. Mary Murphy taught at North Babylon High School as the librarian. Our paths crossed Mary Murphy's when she developed ALS, Mary died in 2004 after a brief year-long battle. Her good friend and colleague, Barbara Brown, also a physical education teacher met and fell in love with the Ride organization.

"I saw the positive effect the Ride and Chris had on Mary." Barbara said explaining her devotion to the organization.

She appreciated and valued the contributions it made in the lives of PALS. When Mary died, Barbara signed on as a volunteer. At first, she helped with various projects, choosing the school assembly programs as her prime focus. Barbara served a short stint on the Board of Directors. However, frustration with the slow, procedure-driven meetings upset her. She saw how rapid the progression spreads. It killed a dear friend in a year.

"I have no patience for all the BS that goes on," she confessed when she resigned from the Board.

She had no desire to deal with the necessary procedures and protocols, which take so long. She chafed at bowing to precedent. Idealistic to a fault, she grew impatient with courting business at the expense of action for PALS now. Barbara was a coach, experienced with organizing an effective, action geared team. She expected her team to win the current match, not delay and talk!

Freed from the behind the scenes side of the organizational focus of the Board, she worked when she had time to strengthen and expand the school assembly program. After retiring in 2011, she devoted endless hours advancing the assemblies. Barbara became the school outreach coordinator. The program grew enormously to become the basis of our largest fundraiser.

During the annual Ride, Barbara coordinated the school stops and route itinerary for many years following Kevin's departure. Tens of thousands of students have learned about ALS while raising a million dollars. The largest chunk of the $8 million raised by our organization came from children.

The schools present this money when we visit during our journey across Long Island. Enthusiastic students of all ages donate to help find a cure. For years, Barbara continued as our Pied Piper leading us from school to school across the Island and the city.

An unlikely event occurred in 2017. Remarkably, the Ride celebrated its twentieth anniversary. This was a most unanticipated occurrence, particularly by me! After the first Ride I, along with everyone assumed this was a one-time activity. As the second spring approached following the event, my health remained good. I put another Ride together for 1999. Using my gift of time, I grew it into an annual event and a respected charity.

By the twentieth Ride, the disease did compromise my body but my spirit remained undiminished. We have been riding in the metropolitan area for 16 years. I wanted to make an anniversary return Ride.

"I want to go back to Washington next year," I told everyone. No one was surprised.

"You are still crazy," my wife told me. "I know you can do it. Good luck."

Daunting as the first planning seemed at the time, the recreating it for the twentieth posed monumental challenges. Foremost, I faced the same question as the first: Who will help me?

Richard Iannuzzi learned about ALS as president of his local teacher union in Central Islip. In 2001, one of his members, home and careers teacher Judy Reilly developed ALS. He moved up to serve as president of the state union, New York State United Teachers. His new role enabled him to give significant support to all teachers with ALS. NYSUT joined as a major sponsor. Upon leaving the position a decade later, he became a member of our Board of Directors. He has been hard at work since. Drawing on his teaching experience, I thought of a project for him.

"Dick, will you help Barbara and me with the school assembly program?"

"What do you have in mind?" he asked.

"Become a co-presenter and work with PALS to deliver assemblies," I explained.

"Count me in!" he countered.

With his help, more schools participated. Working with him, we became friends. I knew he had some time available with no young children or other regular responsibilities demanding his attention.

"Would you please consider helping organize the anniversary Ride return to Washington?" I inquired matter-of-factly. I tried soft selling the task.

"Huh," he said, taken by surprise. He was not sure what I meant.

"It is a repeat and much of the work was done already," I assured him. "Besides, we have an organization to help now. Back then there was nothing to assist."

He listened with attention but seemed unconvinced. "I am not sure I could do it," he replied.

"Charlie will also help you and he did it three times," I pitched my best ball last. With this final inducement, I waited for his reaction.

"I don't know. I can give it a try." Dick hesitantly agreed.

"That is good enough for me," I said before he could change his mind. I promised, "We will make it work." Although, Charlie hadn't committed yet.

"Lord, forgive me for telling a white lie. Please guide Charlie so that he will agree to help Dick," I prayed.

Charlie agreed. Work it did. Dick survived the nail-biting episodes of riding without police escorts, seat of the pants planning, on the fly wheelchair changes done in the middle of the road, endless fast food meals, sleepless nights, scheduling deadlines, harrowing traffic, narrow unsafe roads, wheelchair foot-run-overs and biblical rainstorms. The anniversary Ride was a huge success due in large part to Dick.

No recounting of Ride leadership is complete without mentioning the media. Millions on Long Island recognize the ALS Ride for Life due to the excellent media coverage provided by the cable news organization, News 12. Reporter

Greg Cergol covered the story and moved by his experience, he requested additional airtime. He and his videographer Mike Del Giudice wound up meeting us in D.C. to report on our Congressional reception the final day. Cergol earned an Emmy for his feature.

On the first Long Island Ride in 2001, Greg found my schedule. He surprised me along the route. He stood at the side of the road holding the framed certificate accompanying his Emmy Award statue that he received for his story on the Ride.

"I want you to have this, Chris," Greg told me when he rushed out from the side of the road. "It's your story, you should have it."

"Greg, this so special. Are you sure?"

"Absolutely," he said, handing it to me. Today Greg's Emmy certificate proudly adorns my office wall. I look at it every day and remember.

The following year Bob Butler received the assignment and the tradition was born. Bob and Mike reported on the Ride for several years. Bob became a road regular, often spending hours walking alongside me. He wired me with a microphone and got hours of interview material. In the process, he gained a deeper appreciation for life, loss and the value of time. On the streets, I discovered he was a comedian at heart.

"It's hard to pay the bills doing comedy," Bob revealed. He became a reporter and drew a steady paycheck.

In a couple of years, he experienced the loss of ALS patients he came to know through his Ride reporting.

"You should not live with regrets, Bob. Life is too short. I know it's a cliché, but look at the people we have lost." I advised him.

The following spring, he greeted me with big news. "Chris, my wife and I are moving."

"Where to?" I asked expecting a move to a nicer area of the Island.

"California. I am resigning from the station and taking up my true passion, entertainment."

"Well, that's a shocker. I never saw that coming," I said. "I have to give you credit, you took action to pursue your dreams. Kudos to your wife for supporting your decision."

He resumed his birth name, Wiltfong. Bob, wife Jill and their 3 children are happy West Coasters. Sometimes I tune in a TV show and catch him performing in a guest appearance spot on a series or as an actor in a commercial. We stay in contact through the Web. He never stopped supporting us and runs Web based fundraisers.

The longest and most impactful news reporter I worked with is Elizabeth Hashagen. She is now an anchor for the morning news on News 12. When Elizabeth inherited the task of reporting the Ride after Bob, she confessed.

"I had the jitters. You were already a legend around the station. I was a new, young reporter. I was worried about living up to the standards set by Cergol and Butler, both Emmy Award winners for their Ride stories."

"Well, you would never know it from your work," I told her.

Young, energetic and effervescent, Elizabeth rose and exceeded the standard set for her. In fact, she garnered eleven

Emmy Awards, many for her ALS stories. One was for a Ride documentary she made. On my bookcase in our den sits the golden wing Emmy statue Elizabeth gave to me. It is right beside the one News 12 videographer, Mike Del Giudice, gave me when he won for his Ride filming.

Her enthusiasm is not limited to professional work. Beth also served as the Emcee at our annual Honorary Recognition Benefit gala for over a dozen years. For my recent birthday, she hosted the evening.

Her outstanding reporting, filmed by Brian Jingeleski, helped spread the ALS Ride's story near and far. One year, my wife and I did a bucket list cruise to Alaska. We left the ship to do a shore adventure in Juneau. A voice called from behind asking.

"Are you that ALS guy on the news every year?" a fellow traveler called out.

"That's me," I shouted to her. The power of media to reach audiences is extraordinary.

"I watch you all the time on Channel 12 News," she said in excitement.

Each morning I wake up to the news. If it is an early day, I catch Elizabeth and I smile watching her giving the morning news.

I muse, "How would the Ride be if Elizabeth did not make my fight her fight too?" Her contributions are immeasurable. Elizabeth is a powerful, albeit de facto leader.

The years ahead for the Ride are uncertain. New challenges will arise. I will continue to deteriorate. Who knows what will happen?

As I tell the kids at each school assembly, always be optimistic. I trust, new leaders continue to emerge to lead the fight for a cure.

The lesson I learned from this was giants truly stand on the shoulders of others. My success is entirely dependent on so many who embraced my mission. The accolades I receive is really theirs. I couldn't do it without them. It takes an entire village.

The Perfect Chairman

On the heels of my diagnosis came my advocacy work and efforts to raise research money. An acquaintance helped initiate me into the fundraising world. Ray Manzoni's real estate company ran golf outings for the Muscular Dystrophy Association.

Our daughters went to school together and wound up on the tennis team. The two paired up and played doubles. Ray's daughter, Kim worked at a special needs summer camp and learned a little sign language.

"Let's use it to share our strategy when we play," she conspired with Melissa.

They were a sight on the court. It was a mystery to most opponents and the two appeared to be excellent players anticipating one another's moves. They did well and brought the team several match victories. Ray and I sometimes saw each other at matches and cheered our girls together. We became casual friends through the girls.

When Ray found out my illness came under MDA's umbrella of neuromuscular diseases, he wanted to help me. He continued running the golf outing with the MDA but with one requirement.

"I want to continue running the golf outing," he told the MDA representatives, "but with one stipulation: it must become an ALS-focused event." Ray said.

When the ALS Ride started organizing better, we assumed a larger role in running the event. Eventually, we replaced the MDA all together. All the money from the golf outings went straight to ALS Ride for Life.

Parallel to this, I started volunteering with the new Greater New York chapter of the ALS Association. The young group was eager for support. I created a World Series-based raffle style fundraiser for them, targeting businesses and their customers. However, we needed a major return benefit to entice businesses to sign on. Since the Yankees were often World Series contenders, I set my goal: Get a Yankee player involved. This would get businesses involved. It is much easier to think of it than to produce it.

"Do you have any leads that will help me get a Yankee celebrity to participate?" I asked the NY chapter of the ALS Association.

I received a contact from the national ALS Association, which came during a phone conversation.

"We have the name of a prominent labor negotiator lawyer. She handled the bargaining between the player's union and the Yankees during the 1994-95 baseball strike." They informed me, "The lawyer was well-respected and battled a similar neuromuscular disease, Multiple Sclerosis."

"Perfect," I responded. "Surely she will be sympathetic to our cause and help us. Thank you!"

I looked up Marianne McGettigan of Maine—no easy task in 1995. I sent off a letter. In it, I explained I needed a

Yankee player to help with a fund raising campaign revolving around the World Series for the ALS Association Greater New York Chapter. The single obligation for the player was a short evening appearance at an area business. Within days, my phone rang.

She said, "I know the perfect player. I worked closely with him during the strike. He was the player's representative in the bargaining sessions. I think he will help you. "

"That is terrific news," I exclaimed. "What is his name?"

I am a New Yorker, born and bred. The Metropolitan area has a large Jewish population. I lived a few years in Belle Harbor, Queens among a sizable Jewish community. I was accustomed to hearing surnames that were predominately Jewish. I am also not a big baseball fan.

"It is David Cohen," she announced in her Maine accent.

I was thrilled at the prospect. I thought nothing about it. I assumed he was just another New Yorker who happened to be Jewish. Little did I know there were only a handful of Jewish Yankees players through the years and none from recent times.

While I was on vacation in the Outer Banks, North Carolina, I called his manager as McGettigan had advised, Andrew Levy of Wish You Were Here Productions. My friends, all serious sports fans, gathered around the phone to hear my conversation with a Yankee baseball player's manager.

"Damn it," I shouted when a message machine clicked. I left my message about the campaign details. I requested a player and hoped David Cohen would agree. As I did they burst out in laughter.

One, Kenny Balslov, roared at me, "You knuckle head! If you want a player to help, you better say his name right." I turned as white as the beach sand just beyond the door.

"What?" I asked dumbfounded. "You mean I said his name wrong?"

I slumped, turning from white to red as they ribbed me more. "His name is Cone, not Cohen!" my friend continued, instructing me in baseball 101. Then he added in a serious tone, "You probably just blew your chance."

Bummed out at my stupidity, I left the room.

Several days after I got back home, Andrew Levy called for further information.

"I apologize for my embarrassing error, I did not hear the name clearly," I said to Andrew.

He was unfazed by my naivety brushing it off.

He told me, "I think this might appeal to David. Let me talk with him. I'll be in touch."

Encouraged by the call, I proceeded planning the details for the baseball campaign. I ordered small paper baseballs to sell at participating businesses. The customers sign them and then the business displays them around the walls. The last missing piece was the celebrity "prize" benefit for the business with the highest sales.

We received an answer through a phone call from Andrew.

"Yes! David will do it."

I began printing the promotional flyers, *Have a Yankee Night with David Cone, buy a baseball and Strike Out ALS!* The fundraiser went well.

A large sports complex in Suffolk County sold the most baseballs and won an appearance by David. I went beforehand to check their preparations. The complex roped off a large open space and lines formed before I arrived. The fans held balls, cards, hats and other memorabilia to sign. Excitement flowed and time flew. David's limousine arrived late because it was stuck in traffic coming from Manhattan.

Other than knowing about his famous teammate, Lou Gehrig and Catfish Hunter, David was unfamiliar with ALS. He never met a patient before. I invited a patient to meet David. John Rather, a lawyer from the Island. John was quite progressed. He had a tracheotomy, was quadriplegic and unable to speak. He blinked to communicate. He sat in a large, motorized wheelchair. He presented an imposing and intimidating sight to unsuspecting observers.

"David, I have a patient I want you to meet," I told him. "You can see the effects of this disease. You will understand why we are doing the fundraiser."

I brought David over to greet John in private before the signing session. I studied David's reaction. He appeared taken back. Like a young boy meeting a beautiful girl, he stared not knowing where to look. The sight seemed to take the breath away from David while John's ventilator whirled, pushing breath into him.

David spoke with John, asking customary questions which John answered with a blink. I explained to David.

"John can only reply to yes or no questions," I said to him.

David tried to rephrase some of his queries in the form of yes / no but like most people, found the exchange challenging. I interpreted John's blinking responses. When patience loose speech, many resort to a system of blinks to communicate. It is a tedious, arduous and slow method, one I knew I must use one day.

After the powerful meeting, David smiled and signed autographs for adoring fans waiting for him in the gathering area. It was a memorable evening for the fans and David as well.

The baseball campaign lasted a few years and raised a modest amount. I do not remember the exact amount but around twenty thousand for the New York chapter. Through the campaign, Andrew, David and I grew closer. David's career with the Yankees soared. An award-winning pitcher, David secured his place in baseball lore on July 18, 1999. David became the 16th pitcher to pitch a perfect game. Twenty-seven batters came to plate and twenty-seven were retired. He allowed no runs, no hits and no walks. His pitching was perfect.

As David's career rose, my frustration rose also and my health declined. I had to explain my disease everywhere I went. It was almost unknown. Resources were sparse. The Internet was in its infancy. I owned an Apple computer with a monochrome green display. I used a dial-up phone line for Net access and it was snail slow.

My first contact with other patients came in a Prodigy chat room for ALS patients. Prodigy was a pioneer service provider, long before AOL. We shared stories, supported each other and spoke about the lack of awareness or commitment to finding a cure. I did a crude search with the limited capabilities of the Net at that time.

I typed the initials, ALS. After ten long minutes of waiting, my response came. The search yielded only one site. It was a high-energy physics facility in Germany called the

Alternating Light Synchrotron. Absolutely nothing about the disease. Today, if you type ALS in, hundreds or more sites appear. Back then, it was as if ALS was a phantom disease.

Research lagged well behind diseases that had similar incidence of diagnoses. The National Institute of Health funded all major research. ALS was a tiny blip on their radar. At the rate of funding, ALS, discovered 150 years ago, would take another one hundred years to cure.

It was time to end the benign neglect. If patients and their families did not lead the way, who would? Some vowed to fight for our own lives. The organizers appropriately called our loose knit group PROD, a play on the server name of Prodigy. The goal was advocacy, push patients into action. I took the name, 'Stop ALS.' The members were the unsung heroes who began the advocacy movement, sadly their names long forgotten. Jack Norton and Ted Hein were two giants leading the charge. With PROD, the era of advocacy began. It altered the history of ALS. They motivated me to do my part.

My ALSA GNY paper baseball campaign with David continued for several more years. I appeared on the Jerry Lewis MDA Telethon, a Labor Day weekend TV tradition for decades. In 1995, I was invited to testify before a subcommittee of the Federal Drug Administration to push for the approval of an experimental drug for ALS.

"We demand the approval of Rilutek," I stated to the subcommittee during the hearing. "It is the first drug clinically proven to help patients. It may have only a modest benefit of a three-month extension of life," I continued, "Three months may mean a daughter's wedding, a college graduation or a family reunion. You must not deny a dying person that gift! Approve the drug."

During the gathering, many advocates demonstrated outside the FDA headquarters. The building fronted a major highway. The sides of the property facing the road were sloped. We stood on the crest and waved signs. I stumbled on the uneven ground; I fell and tumbled down the incline into the street. People ran from everywhere to block traffic. I laid there unable to get up. Someone called the police about a protester laying in the road stopping traffic. In pain, I sprawled out and waited until help came. The road temporarily closed. The crowd cheered and clapped as they chanted slogans. They thought I intentionally laid down to stop traffic.

A handful of police cars pulled up from all directions. They jumped out ready to clear the street of protesters. My wife explained the situation to the police when they approached me lying across a lane in the road. The arrest mode morphed into an aid call.

"Are you okay?" the officer asked.

"Yes, just a bit sore and dizzy," I answered.

Satisfied I didn't require an ambulance and was not intentionally blocking the road in protest, they assisted me to my feet. The police officers helped me walk off the road.

The crowd clamored their support. I was the hero of the day for putting my life on the line for ALS.

"Thanks but I really don't deserve credit. Blame my bum legs and the sloping side shoulder." I told the group. Even with my explanation, they continued anyway.

I received the reputation as the person who laid in the road and blocked traffic. Both the testimony and the demonstration whetted my thirst to do more public advocacy. I had to continue my momentum. There was work do. I started planning the ALS Ride for Life four years after my diagnosis in 1993. I rode my wheelchair to Washington in 1998 to galvanize patients and inform the public.

For the second Ride in 1999, I asked David Cone to send us off from the Stadium. He agreed. The news featured Yankee pitcher David Cone cutting the ribbon in front of the Stadium to start the Ride.

For the fourth Ride in 2001 came the new venue and more opportunities. More than ever, the organization needed a well-known face to represent us. Again, I thought David might help.

"Would David consider becoming our honorary spokesperson?" I asked Andrew.

"I'll speak to him and let you know," Andrew said.

We got our answer. With pride, our next brochure featured the expression, "Join my team and strike out ALS," along with David's photo pitching. Today he continues to serve as our Honorary Chairman. The number of events and activities David did is amazing.

He was the right choice to be our honorary chair.

In fact, David Cone is the 'Perfect' Chairman in every way.

The lesson I learned from this was sports celebrities are powerful allies, which add such credibility and influence to an organization. The ALS Ride for Life was fortunate to have the support of David Cone and Andrew Levy.

Catch

I tried to make a case that ALS, although uncommon, was far from rare. For a long time, I searched for a way to make the dimension of ALS tangible to unaware Americans. Large numbers exceed our ability to visualize beyond being "big." It gets lost as an abstraction. Just as a young child thinks of a year and a decade with the same incomprehension, adults think similarly of large numbers. In order to drive home the scale of the dying, I needed to think of some concrete illustration. How could I represent the number of lives lost yearly? Without a visual, the magnitude would remain an abstraction, and ALS patients would continue to suffer neglect.

There was so much work remaining. By 2006, I was speaking about ALS whenever I could. I met Brie, a St. Joseph's College student, during her internship at Channel 12 News. She worked on the news coverage of the Ride. When she returned to school the next semester, Brie wanted to help the Ride.

"Will you speak to my class about being a disabled person overcoming obstacles? This would be good for my classmates. Many will work with that population," Brie asked me.

"Of course. Set it up and I'll be there," I answered.

She was a Recreation major and wanted me sharing experiences as a disabled person. Her professor, Dr. Gail Lamberta was supportive.

The college is a small commuter school. She waited for me in the parking lot and escorted me to the room. Traveling across campus, we passed an art department exhibit called 'Kinetic Art'.

"Check that out," calling her attention to the display by the art department.

I prefer realistic examples of art such as paintings of landscape, portraits and nature photography. I found the display, honestly, rather silly. The whole exhibit was nothing more than pinwheels randomly placed in the green commons.

"Humph," she said not focusing. Her thoughts were on her introduction comments.

A waste, I thought keeping my ideas to myself. It was typical of crazy artists. How I came to take back those thoughts....

I did not know at the time but I found my answer to represent the dimension of ALS deaths. I had my concrete illustration. While daydreaming in my wheelchair, I thought of something in my youth. It was a Dylan Thomas song, "Blowing in the Wind."

Pinwheels are relatively cheap, durable for an outdoor display and visually appealing. Synergistically, I linked the two ideas. The cure is out there somewhere blowing around in the wind. Pinwheels catch it, spinning when it does. I melded the song's meaning of answers in the wind and the pinwheels. I created a new song expressing the pain, suffering and hope of ALS.

How many roads must a man wheel down
Before you call him a man?
How many seas must a white dove sail
Before she sleeps in the sand?
How many times must the cannonballs fly
Before they're forever banned?
The answer, my friend, is blowing' in the wind
The answer is blowing' in the wind

How many years must we wait for a cure
While too many people die?
How many tears must we wipe from our eyes
While ALS keeps taking lives?
How many times can a man turn his head
Pretending he just doesn't see?
The answer, my friend, is blowing' in the wind
The answer is blowing' in the wind

How many times must a man look up
Before he can see the sky?
How many ears must one man have
Before he can hear patients cry?
How many deaths will it take till he knows
That too many people have died?
The answer, my friend, is blowing' in the wind
The answer is blowing' in the wind

The cure for ALS is blowing somewhere in the wind. We must catch it, the same as the pinwheels catch the wind. Thank you, Brie and St. Joseph's Art department. I especially want to thank Dr. Lamberta, because she maintained the connection Brie began. St Joseph's remains involved to this day. I went to work to get six thousand pinwheels to use for the 2007 Ride.

Don Strasser started the student club at Northport High School called, *A Mid Winter's Night Dream,* to support his friend and colleague, David Deutsch. He was the second teacher in the district diagnosed with ALS at the same time as I was. Between David and myself, almost every student in the high school knew one of us.

"Don, would your students put up six thousand pinwheels at Columbia University?" I sheepishly asked him.

"I'll try to make it happen," he answered. "There are a lot of problems we need to work out, but I want to help Dave and you."

Early in the morning hours on the last day of that Ride, sleepy students from the club and Don piled on a school bus and drove to Gehrig's alma mater, Columbia University. Don's students were hard at work erecting pinwheels in the large rectangular Central Mall in front of the University library before we arrived to end the last day. They finished moments ahead of our arrival. David died in 2012. The club went on to raise several million dollars to fight ALS before disbanding in 2017.

We rolled into campus to the evocative sight of 6,000 whirling, murmuring pinwheels. Each new breeze stirred them anew. They sung as if they were the voices of our fallen patient Riders.

"Remember us, keep riding, don't give up, find the cure," they wailed.

The sight was stunning and sobering. My dark humor forced me to say, "The sight stole your breath away. " Except of course, for patients who maintained theirs because of their ventilator.

It moved everyone who saw it. Most cried at the sight. If they didn't, they did with the ending. Ashley Flanagan, a former Habitat Helper and now Broadway actor, closed the day by her exquisite rendering of *Amazing Grace*.

Thanks to President Stanley and Vice President Kaushansky, the pinwheel display has found a permanent home at Stony Brook University. Each May pinwheels go up in a Field of Hope on campus to celebrate ALS Awareness Month. The tedious geometric arrangement is a time-consuming ritual coordinated by university staffer, Stuart Campbell. Greek Organizations on campus, local businesses, scouts and school groups, along with Ride volunteers assist. On their way to the university, thousands of motorists see the glittering metallic silver and red wheels spinning in waves from the breeze moving across the meadow.

They spin to remind us, the cure is out there, blowing in the wind. All we need to do is catch it.

The lesson I learned from this was great ideas may originate from unusual sources. Be open to things and don't be too quick to pass judgment. As the saying goes, "minds are like parachute. They only work well when they are open."

A Road Not Taken

ALS Ride 2013 remained months away. My decision was spontaneous.

"Christine, what do you think of a new route for Port Jefferson to Stony Brook," I asked my wife.

After years of following one route through Port Jefferson Station, we decided to change the roads for this segment. The new direction brought us through the village of Port Jefferson. I reasoned that it was more hometown and would provide greater opportunity to spread awareness. It was a much more pleasant route making it more attractive for walkers to join us. Although others questioned the break with tradition, I felt comfortable with the new plan.

In no time, the day of the Ride arrived. The morning began with threatening dark skies and a cool breeze. Forecasts called for rain.

"Do we stop in the rain?" asked a walker joining us for the day after looking at the sky.

"Does ALS stop killing during inclement weather?" I replied.

"No."

"Then, we don't stop fighting it, even in the rain."

Undeterred, we wheeled off from our starting point at an Empire National Bank branch, in Port Jefferson Station.

The bank is a great community business and a generous supporter. The divided highway contained the normal heavy traffic of a Saturday morning. Other patients with ALS, Steve DePasquale in his chair, Paul Weissman who walked and I rolled along behind the police escort. A gaggle of supporters brought up the rear.

The spectacle of such an entourage traveling down the road achieved its goal as everyone slowed down to investigate the peculiar parade. The huge, trailer borne sign, sixteen feet long, and ten feet in the air proclaimed "Strike Out ALS." We were spreading awareness, for sure!

My eye caught a red figure off in the distance. On the opposite side of the divider, a red shirted woman emerged.

"Chris! Chris!" she called.

Amid the other commotion and craziness, this occurrence did not strike me as unusual. Over the years and through extensive media coverage, I had become a well- known figure in the community. I assumed the woman was another excited bystander who recognized me.

I smiled and nodded as I passed. She waved and shouted, but I did not pick up on her message. I could not read her T-shirt she was pointing out. At 64, my ears and eyes are not what they were. Unaware, I continued riding.

My wife who was walking in the back, did recognize her (in my defense, my wife does wear glasses!). At the next intersection, our group turned off the highway heading toward the village. Breathless, my wife caught up with me and told me the surprising news.

She said, "That woman in the red shirt was Vinnie Cullen's assistant."

Three months earlier, I heard about a new patient whom I must meet, Vinnie Cullen. He was a fighter and go-getter. Finally, I thought, perhaps another patient like me. Someone I hoped who would work beside me to help tame the beast afflicting us. I made an appointment to meet in his office.

I rolled into the room saying, "Hey Vinnie, nice to meet you."

He greeted me with a broad smile, vigorous head nodding and thumbs up. The disease already stole Vinnie's voice.

Vinnie was able to scribble his thoughts. His assistant of 16 years, Karen facilitated most of our conversation. Sometimes she did not even need to wait for him to finish writing because she intuitively knew what he wanted to say. We plotted and planned. He agreed to get involved with no hesitation.

"I can make some connections among school districts across the island," he said through Karen.

He was a CPA auditor and knew many key administrators from doing financial reviews of school districts. His recommendations would allow us to get into some more schools to do the assembly program. We waxed about advocacy and the upcoming Ride.

"I am looking forward to riding with you Chris," he told me.

"Well Vinnie, I am very happy to have a new companion. The more, the merrier!"

Two months before the Ride, we held a kickoff celebration, the Honoree Recognition Benefit. I anticipated introducing him that evening to his new family of Ride supporters. ALS had other plans for us. Vinnie took a nasty fall attempting to get dressed to come. Badly bruised and banged up, he never made it.

Following his fall, the emails became less frequent. Karen shared that Vinnie was failing fast. I attempted to rally him in emails by referencing the great time to come. Participating in the Ride was life altering for a patient. Diagnosis often left patients devoid of hope. I knew a Ride For Life experience restores it.

"My husband, Larry Lefkowitz lives in a nursing facility because he is trached. He all but gave up on living," his distraught wife Florence explained. "I wanted him home, but I couldn't." she apologized for her inability to do what is a daunting task, caring for a PALS on a trache. She asked me to visit him and give him encouragement.

I went to visit him. We spoke about the challenges he faced. He enjoyed hearing the history of the Ride.

"The Ride will be recognized by the Yankees at a home plate ceremony," I enticed him. I knew he was a rabid fan. His eyes widened and sparkled with interest.

"You want to join me?" I asked.

The trach made talking difficult. The air-filled cuff, which anchored the tube in his windpipe blocked airflow over his vocal chords. Occasionally, the cuff could deflate for short periods, allowing speech. Most of the time he mouthed simple phrases.

"Are you kidding?" he mouthed to me. He lit up like a lighthouse.

"Of course not. I am serious," I assured him.

"How?" he asked.

I advocated for PALS to be mobile. I fought for his right to travel beyond the walls of his facility. Florence pushed for her husband. The facility acquiesced. The Ride paid for a respiratory therapist and transportation. Larry appeared with me and other supporters at home plate.

"You gave me a reason to live," he told me in tears as we rolled toward home plate.

Participating in the Ride wins back a sense of purpose and empowerment stripped away by the paralyzing disease. I knew doing the Ride would be the best medicine Vinnie could have. The same effect it demonstrated with Larry so many years ago.

I tried to focus on Christine's words, which were coming rapid fire. Sitting in the middle of the street at a traffic light was not the ideal spot for a conversation. It was difficult for me to concentrate. Her words began to make sense. It dawned on me and the fog lifted. The woman was not an admiring bystander I realized. It was Vinnie's assistant, Karen. She was not shouting encouragement, but was trying to tell me something. I misunderstood.

"Three days before the Ride began, Vinnie passed away." My wife informed me.

Now I had the explanation for his no show for the Ride this morning. Like with the HRB event a couple of months earlier, ALS had other plans for Vinnie. It killed him before he could join other patients on his Ride For Life. Traveling further without my expected new partner made me quite sad. I was on his home turf in Port Jefferson and his absence hurt. He should have been with me that day.

"Damn you, ALS," I screamed into the chilly, wet wind.

What Christine shared next was not believable. Vinnie's wake was *today and right down* the block. Christine was involved in almost every aspect of the Ride planning. We made this route change together. Because of it, we were now going right by there on our way to the village. My wife and I looked at each other.

After 40 years of marriage, we know each other's thoughts. So, this was the reason? The route plan was for Vinnie. It was done months ago without us realizing. In death, he *was* able to beat ALS. He defied the damn disease for once. He would be on the Ride.

I pictured Vinnie singing Frank Sinatra's song, "I did it my way."

As we neared the funeral home, we outlined a new plan to the police. When they heard about the reason for the change they were happy to accommodate.

"Follow the lead police car. He will escort you into the funeral home's circular driveway," the unit supervisor said.

We gathered at Vinnie's side, even though separated by the building's wall. That did not matter. We were together. Vinnie could not come to us, so we came to him. Vinnie made the Ride. He got his wish, although not the way all of us wanted.

In the book of Jeremiah, it says, "I know, O LORD, that a man's way is not his own; no one who walks directs his own steps."

Still, I say he beat ALS and got his way for a change. The Ride took a Road Not Taken and Vinnie was on it.

The lesson I learned from this was victory comes in a variety of ways. Sometimes, it comes in a way we did not want and be bittersweet.

Planning Ahead

The myriad of details required by the Ride boggles the mind. In many respects, current Ride preparations dwarf those of the early D.C. days. In addition, there were the two big weekend public participation days. It was enough to keep a small army of staff occupied. For the most part, we did it through volunteers.

Following the adage, "The squeaky wheel gets the oil," the priority issues were resolved first. We tackled tasks in sequence of when they occurred. Since the Ride began on a Monday, planning tasks needed for a Saturday seemed an eternity away. We put those requirements on the back burner. Another reason to postpone those tasks, there were no schools involved.

Coordinating with school schedules was very trying at best. The response time was long. Teachers were in class all day. By days end they wanted to get home. It frustrated our school coordinator and held up other details.

"Barbara, hound them until they get sick and tired of being pestered and then they will respond," I told her.

Saturday planning was relatively easy and straightforward. I pushed away those items to handle the more pressing, immediate demands. By the time most of our weekday planning was complete, the Ride was about to begin.

Way behind schedule, I turned my attention to figuring out logistics for the first Saturday. Many holes remained for the day. We had lunch to figure out. An army as well as the Ride moves on its stomach. Naturally, what goes in must come out. Equally important, we needed bathroom facilities.

I went online to contact a local fire department. Its location was ideal, situated half way along the route. I detailed all about the Ride and ended with a simple request.

"Chief, may we stop for lunch at the firehouse and also use the bathrooms?" I said in an email. "All we need is your parking lot for a rest stop. Our group will be about 50."

I felt relieved with the potentially easy fix. In the past, other fire departments helped with similar requests. I was confident it would work. I moved on to other fish to fry. I awaited their response.

Days went by with no news. I was not alarmed because organizations such as the fire department have an irregular schedule and the volunteers are not available. Requests such as mine took time to approve. We solved many of the other requirements. I thought everything was coming together. When my computer screen flashed with an email from the fire department, I eagerly opened it.

"Thank you for your recent email. We regret to inform you, we cannot assist you this year. We have other events planned."

I read it twice to make sure. What disappointing news. We needed a bathroom break and I had few options. Most urgent and difficult was finding bathrooms for a large group. We could eat anywhere. After waiting so long for a reply, there was only a week to go.

We looked and found a church about half way on the route. It had easy road access.

"Thank God," I thought. "Surely they would help us."

I dictated an email to the pastor. Unlike my request to the fire department, I appealed to their faith-based commitment to helping people in need. It was my "Hail Mary pass" because I was desperate. The Methodist Church of Three Village was my last hope.

Again, days went by before I heard from the assistant pastor for youth.

His email said, "The pastor was away and your request was given to me. I want to help. The lateness of your request and my concerns about being able to meet your expectations gives me reservations."

"I assure you we have no expectations except to have a place to safely rest, shelter from the sun and refresh off the road." I answered.

"Then we will be blessed to help."

Plans were complete. Thank you Lord and Mary.

Saturday morning was overcast and threatening. There was a soft mist blowing in the early morning as we arrived at the staging point. As we organized, the walkers knotted in small bunches to talk about the day. Volunteers prepared the mobile sign and coordinated with the police escort, while others gathered the day's supply of water and snacks. The other patient and I donned our bright yellow angler's foul-weather gear: besides protecting us from the weather, it was also an excellent way of standing out as we moved among the traffic along the highway.

On schedule, we all assembled to begin. I tried to put a spin on the weather.

I declared, "It is a brilliant Irish morning for a stroll."

The police pulled out onto the street and we followed the flashing lights of our escort. The hardy group walked through the rain, plodding ahead and clicking off the miles. When we left the harbor downtown, we eyed the imposing hill that lie ahead. Surrounding the sleepy seaside village were large hills formed by glaciers.

"More than 15,000 years ago half mile-high sheets of ice carved these valleys. It formed this hill," I shared with the struggling walkers. I thought diverting their attention might ease the climb.

Half way through the ascent, I secretly welcomed the cool overcast and intermittent drops. Like Edmond Hillary first mounting Everest, our motley crew reached the summit. They were jubilant. Beyond the hill, a mile down the road was the church. Mercifully, it was largely downhill. By the time we reached it, we were bedraggled, exhausted, wet and all in need of refuge. Seven miles were behind but seven more remained in front.

Smiling, cheering and clapping young people from the church youth ministry lined the driveway. Their smiles chased away any clouds. At the head of the line was the young assistant pastor, Rev. Lou Pizzichillo, who greeted us with open arms.

"Come, you made it. Come inside and cool off, rest yourselves. We are happy to have you."

They led us to the door of the church and beseeched us to enter their sanctuary. Gratefully, we obliged. We felt welcomed and warmed.

"Thank you," Christine said.

We settled into a large meeting room dominated by a long, plain table that sat in the center, flanked by chairs along its rim. The corners had stuff piled up, like car hulks stored in an auto salvage yard. The congregation swarmed over us tending to our every need. The food spread looked like a gourmet's feast.

"Please, help yourself," one of the church youth ministry bid us.

The young people, thirsty for knowledge, questioned the participants about ALS and why they chose to walk. Chatter and fellowship filled the room and an air of belonging wafted over us.

Savoring the blessing that was unfolding before me, my eyes scanned the room. In the corner next to me, I spied a dry erase white board with notes on it. Curious, I squinted to decipher the words. To my surprise, I discovered what I assumed were lecture notes the youth minister used to prep teenagers about our visit. I was impressed.

I thought, "Goodness, he went the extra mile to counsel them about us and what to expect."

As I read the disjointed phrases, my mind's eye could see his talk unfolding. He added each new point with an additional phrase on the white board. Even though the minister never met us, or anyone with ALS, the phrases he chose were right on target.

"I hit pay dirt with this find," I thought. It helped me compose my thank you comments.

My admiration and appreciation for him, the congregation and the church continued to grow. I could not envision a warmer, more hospitable setting for our lunch stop. It was, well, heaven!

Time raced and we needed to return to the road. Miles of pavement remained and we were on a tight schedule. Far too soon, we prepared to part our new friends. Wanting to thank them, I decided to focus my words on the whiteboard. Before speaking, I employed the time-tested strategy of finding out who my audience was and their background.

I began by innocently asking, "What was that white board shoved up against the corner?"

Taken off guard, the minister shrugged his shoulders, motioning ignorance with his facial and body language. He turned to some of the deacons in the group and asked them if they knew anything about the white board. A hand raised and a young man spoke.

"I believe it was written by my father when he was active in the church ministries." The man continued, "Since my father is no longer here, we stuck it in the corner. Nobody knew what to do with it, and I was not going to erase it. So, it has just sort of stayed here, hanging around," he finished, a bewildered look on his face.

"When did your dad do that?" I asked, quite surprised at the revelation.

"I don't know. It's got to be ten years."

The answer stunned me. I thought it was written just days earlier. I incorrectly assumed the youth minister wrote it to prepare the students for our arrival. Yet, it was a decade old. I could not escape the undeniable correlation. The six phrases were tailor made for us today.

It perfectly presaged the morning's events. I read each of the six phrases to everyone. I added how they tied in with us today.

Push through the fog - exactly what we had done on that misty, overcast morning. We pushed because there was no other option, except to give up and no one was willing.

We have a disability - the patients profoundly disabled by the progressive paralysis of ALS. However, whether it shows or is hidden, everyone is disabled in some capacity.

We are weak - after trudging seven miles up and down hills the group arrived spent.

We come in Jesus' name—I explained my "Hail Mary pass" email to the pastor. I mentioned how I referenced Joseph and Mary seeking a place to rest while she carried Jesus. "I was a stranger and you invited me in…"

We come as we are - our group was composed of the family, friends, and supporters of patients. Humbled by hope, we were simple people. We came as we were.

I can rest in His Love - believing and invoking Psalm 23, He will provide and in His Love, you will find rest. You demonstrated the love of Jesus.

When I was done, everyone sat silent in contemplation.

"How could it be written ten years ago?" they all wondered.

The real plans were years old. Perhaps my last minute appeal was not so last minute after all. Maybe it was not belated as I thought, but right on *His* schedule. With human hubris, I used my schedule but I was on God's schedule.

For many years, Three Village Church continued to welcome us to their sanctuary.

I guess I should put more faith into the phrase, "Man plans, but God decides."

The lesson I learned from this was there are mysterious coincidences in life. Some consider them luck. I believe there is a plan behind it. I think God decides and we plan. Sometimes they coincide.

Where There Is Smoke

My wife, caregiver, Rose, and I were returning from western Nassau County two days before the end of the 2013 Ride. A mile from home, my wife slowed for a traffic light ahead. We were exhausted from the cumulative effects of the many hours on the road for the last ten days. Our van slowed near the red light. We were unaware of the looming vehicle racing toward us from behind.

A massive pulse of energy and explosive sound enveloped us. It felt like a bomb blew under the van. A horrendous grinding, scraping and vibrating gripped the van. I can feel the movement even now when I think about it. My eyes clamped shut.

"God, when will this end?" I begged, "Please let it be soon." I tried to muster courage telling myself, "Just hang in there."

The speeding car rear-ended our van. The impact pushed us forward into the other lane. The groaning van silenced when it finally stopped dragging across the pavement. It came to a rest and it ended. There was an eerie silence.

The van remained upright. I stared at the roof strapped into my chair. My feet pointed up in the air with my head tilted on a downward angle. My head dangled in pain because the impact knocked it off the headrest. Disoriented, dazed and confused, I struggled to make sense of the chaos.

"Why am I in this awkward, uncomfortable position?" I asked knowing no one would hear.

The crash ripped my ventilator mask to the side but I was still able to breathe through it. My leg ached. I was not able to move my head enough to see what happened. Growing more aware, I realized my mouth was bleeding. My tongue brushed against small objects that filled my mouth. I assumed I knocked out some teeth. I spit them out.

The incessant screaming of Rose finally got my attention. She was standing, looking down at me.

Hysterical, she repeatedly shouted. "Chris, Chris, Chris!" over and over.

Ignoring her, I glanced forward as best I could. I saw my wife's face looking down at me.

I heard her shaking yet reassuring voice say several times, "It's okay, we're okay."

I asked, "What is wrong with my mouth? She studied the mixture of blood and spit. "Are they teeth?" I wanted to know.

"No, they are not teeth. They're chips of glass," she said. The large window beside me shattered.

Refocusing on Rose, I told her, "I am okay!"

"No you are NOT!" she screamed, sobbing.

Already understanding much of what happened and feeling battered, but sound, I told her, "Yes, I am." I tried to calm her.

In the background, I heard Christine was on the phone with a 911 operator. Rose calmed, gathering her composure.

She adjusted my ventilator mask and held my head up so I could breathe easier.

Moments raced. The firehouse was half a mile down the road. In no time, I heard the sirens signaling relief was on its way. The rear lift gate I use to get in and out of the van was smashed. Like a wild animal, I was trapped in a steel cage. A handful of firefighters clamored into the van through the side door. The tremendous force of the crash had snapped the stainless steel rod controlling my chair-tilting mechanism. They looked in bewilderment at my position-thrust into the air backward. They saw Rose holding my head upright and the vent mask.

This was not going be a routine extraction. Through-out the year these First Responders train for situations like this. They assessed my condition and planned my exit. Suddenly, the interior of the van filled with dense, pungent smoke. For the first time since it all began, I panicked.

"God help us, we were on fire!" I thought.

The heavy smoke elevated the call from an extraction to a rescue. The firefighters raced to get me out right away. Four men surrounded me and stretched as if they were playing a game of *Twister* in order to get a good grip on my chair bottom. With super human strength sometimes seen in a crisis, they managed to drag the 625-pound combined weight of the heavy wheelchair and me across the floor to the side door. With a collective grunt, they lifted me up and out of the van. They carried me a short distance to safety.

I thought I would burn to death strapped helpless in the van. Thank God for the first responders of Mt. Sinai Fire Department to whom I am forever grateful.

They put me on a backboard, secured my head and arms. On the way to the ambulance, they walked beside me holding my ventilator. Before we took off, several minutes passed. Those around the van saw the smoke subside as suddenly as it began.

"The smoke was not caused by a fire!" they stated in puzzlement.

I knew in an instant what happened. By accident in the tight quarters and confusion, someone hit a switch turning on my chair. In the commotion, nobody noticed my wheels were spinning rapidly in place. The tires grew red hot and began melting the thin rubber mat underneath. I was like a teenager doing wheelies with their parent's car. I caused the billowing smoke.

That morning before we left John Johnson, my friend from upstate labored an hour in the humid early morning air. He untangled and repositioned my tie-down straps. During the previous two weeks, they had become a knotted nightmare, looking more like a plate of spaghetti than safety straps. They could not tighten anymore. Frustrated, I used only two of the four.

In the past, I often teased John about his compulsive focus on neatness and order. His fastidiousness kept me locked in place during the accident. Otherwise, I think I would have hurled forward to my death.

"John, you saved my life!" I told him.

At the hospital, Christine, Rose and I were all treated and released. I suffered some cuts from the glass window and on my leg along with some sprains from tossing around in the chair, nothing serious. The others fared better. Rose went for some physical therapy on her back. Christine had some aches from the air bags. Pretty damn lucky I'd say. I chose not to sue the older gentleman who hit us. We got our payment already: no one was seriously hurt!

I was also grateful about the van. At first, the body shop told us the damage was beyond fixing. Insurance would not consider the additional value of the $5,000 handicap lift because it was not original. They would only pay the market amount of the van itself.

"It is a 14-year-old van and the market value is insufficient to justify repair," he thought.

We were sickened at the news because we had borrowed the van from a fellow patient, Steve Depasquale. He and wife Susie received it as a loaner van from the Ride for Life and they depended on it. One of our missions is to help patients through loaner equipment like handicap vans. This vital service helps families deal with one of the many burdens and the expenses of ALS. Non-disabled people do not understand the importance of a handicap van. It represents the priceless gift of freedom. It allows access to the world and gives wheelchair dependent people a lifeline to living.

Now, I destroyed it for Steve and felt terrible. However, the final decision rested with an adjuster from the insurance company. We waited, prayed and hoped. Then we received stunning news.

"Mr. Pendergast, the insurance authorized the repairs," the body shop told me.

The van would be repaired. It was a small miracle, thank you Lord. It was the perfect ending to a horrible experience.

We accepted God's grace and thought no more about it. After repairs, it returned to the patient.

Soon after, my wife happened to talk with Denny Leung, the husband of Kim, a deceased patient participant from past Rides. Denny said he was at the same body shop and by chance met our insurance adjuster. He saw the van and struck up a conversation with the adjuster. Denny related the exchange.

"I recognized the name," the adjuster told Denny. "He was my daughter's teacher."

Denny went on to give the adjuster's name, which I am keeping anonymous to protect his identity. When my wife filled me in on the story details, I was awed.

The adjuster was a parent from Dickinson Elementary School where I taught. His daughter was a student for three years in my Habitat Helper program. We had a wonderful relationship. His daughter was a committed and capable assistant helping care for the animal collection. It became a family affair and they took our chinchillas home on long weekends and summer vacation. He and his wife also worked on special projects. He helped with heavy jobs that I no longer could handle. Their special needs son loved spending time with the animals and visited often. His daughter went on to become a "Chinchilla" expert and bred her own. It was a win for both them and me.

Years later, the adjuster saw an opportunity to pay it forward and help ALS patients and me. I believe he found a way to make the van repairable. The work was well beyond the value of the vehicle. He never told me about anything. I guess he preferred to remain anonymous. If it were not for Denny, I would've never known.

I found out the saying, "where there is smoke, there is fire" is not always true. Sometimes there may be something else at work far more awesome than fire.

God is good. He works in mysterious but wonderful ways.

Some will say these events had nothing to do with God. They were random happenings. I think otherwise. I say, thank you, amen.

The lift eventually became unrepairable because parts were no longer available. The van has since been retired from the Ride for Life program. It's probably still serving someone, somewhere.

The lesson I learned from this was it pays to take the time to fix things when they require repair. Sometimes it takes a fastidious person to insist on things working correctly. Thank goodness we have them among us.

A Child Shall Lead Them

As an educator, I am proud of the role of children changing the world, one-step at a time. Through the years, students have played a part in many campaigns to solve significant problems for which they feel passion. Later generations often forget these accomplishments.

For example, more than a half a century ago, a generation of committed and compassionate schoolchildren led the way to curing the scourge of polio. The first significant polio epidemic took place in 1916. The disease grew steadily, reaching a record in 1952 with nearly 60,000 cases. During the 1930s, concerns mounted. Public pools were closed, large events canceled and neighborhood parks were empty. Parents were terrified for their children because polio was highly contagious.

A year after he was sworn in for a second term, Franklin Roosevelt, a 1921 polio victim, responded to the growing pressure to end the menacing illness. On January 3, 1939, he formed an organization to combat Polio, fund research and find a cure. The group received popular support among radio and movie personalities. The well-known entertainer and actor Eddie Cantor lent his support.

Cantor promoted a nationwide campaign to celebrate the upcoming birthday of the President at the end of January by helping him raise money, ten cents at a time. He nicknamed his effort to celebrate Roosevelt's birthday "The March of Dimes."

In his weekly radio address, an elated Roosevelt revealed the results. About 100,000 letters poured into the White House in the two days prior to his birthday. The letters contained change, mostly dimes sent by children. In total, $85,000 was raised, a major portion from students across the country.

The organization turned the successful appeal into an annual Christmas campaign. The March of Dimes against polio was born. Every Christmas, the organization sent letters along with a card containing slots for dimes. The letter encouraged children to put in dimes (a dime at that time was worth $1.75 when adjusted for inflation). Sidewalk booths were set up everywhere, especially near stores. They asked children to drop a dime in the slot. The children's response was overwhelming. The campaign collected an estimated 7 billion dimes before Salk developed the polio vaccine in 1955.

In another case, as scientists battled polio, architects worked to solve other challenges in the country. The island of Manhattan was choking due to the lack of easy and rapid access to the mainland. It was isolated on the west by a wide and formidable river. In 1931, engineers erected the longest suspension bridge in the world across the Hudson River. It stretched from New York City to New Jersey almost a mile away. The high bridge lights were visible up and down the river making the lighthouse standing at its base obsolete. A popular children's book from 1942, *The Little Red Lighthouse and the Great Grey Bridge*, immortalized the plight of the small lighthouse standing under the massive steel bridge.

The book endeared the bridge to children everywhere by its heartwarming portrayal of the lighthouse's plight. The news that the U.S. Coast Guard planned to sell the unnecessary lighthouse for scrap metal caused an uproar. In particular, city students identified with the book. They wrote letters to save their beloved building. After a massive effort, the children pressured the Coast Guard to deed it to New York City. A New York City Park surrounds the lighthouse under the towering bridge today as a symbol of determination and power of children united for a purpose.

A third student intervention took place around the same period. It involved America's premier poet, Walt Whitman. His 1819 birthplace, a long neglected primitive farmhouse, sat on valuable suburban land in Huntington Station, Long Island, New York along an arterial business corridor. Non-descendant owners wanted to sell it to developers. An outcry arose and attempts to preserve it began in earnest.

A group called The Walt Whitman Birthplace Association formed in 1949 and agreed on a price of $20,000 to purchase the site. They had two years to raise the money. One month before the deadline, they were still $10,000 short. The Association turned to Alicia Patterson, founder and publisher of Newsday, the nation's largest suburban newspaper for assistance.

After the paper ran the story on its front page, public support mushroomed, led by Long Island students. Newsday mounted a vigorous campaign for donations. Area schools responded and pennies, nickels, dimes and quarters came pouring in to the Association. A school club, Culluloo, from the Valley Stream Junior High School, led the donors with

$1,300. The Association purchased the site with the money raised. All within the month's deadline,

Today Whitman's birthplace is a New York State Historic Site and on the United States National Register of Historic Places. It was one month away from a bulldozer. Instead, classes of students visit the site every day to enjoy and learn at the restored poet's home. Kids enjoy it today because other students before them cared enough to act.

In similar fashion, I too wanted to galvanize schoolchildren everywhere to rise above "challenges and defy the odds." I wanted to make them an integral part of the process to cure ALS. When the Ride switched to the metro area, I got my opportunity.

Jerome Shor taught Spanish and advised the Junior Honor Society at my district's high school. One of my former students, Naomi Edlin, was one of his students.

"Mr. Shor, you should invite Mr. Pendergast to speak to the club," she said.

He liked her idea and invited me. I went and made my first presentation to students. I was anxious and unsure of their reactions.

Jerry told me "The impact was palpable." He advised me, "Do it everywhere."

Thanks to Jerry, I had the inspiration and confidence to begin my school presentations. From the humble origin in 2000, it grew into an acclaimed and well-received program we have today.

At first, I spoke to the students myself, then with an assistant and finally used a co-presenter to deliver much of the script when my voice became weaker. As requests grew for more programs at new schools, I formed teams of other patients from the Ride to help meet the demand. In 2015 I lost the ability to talk clearly enough to present the program and embraced the emerging technology of eye controlled computers and voice synthesizers.

With this amazing innovation, I was able to continue. For the 2017-2018 school year, we delivered over 80 assembly presentations. The program beams a message of hope and illustrates the ability to not only meet but also overcome life's challenges. I use the Iron Horse of baseball, Lou Gehrig, and my multi-year battle with ALS, as models of determination and perseverance for students to follow. Like the Ride itself, the assembly program was 'home grown' in my own Northport School District.

The first few Rides on the Island were similar to the D.C. trips: the focus was on public awareness. We started at the Montauk Lighthouse at the very tip of Long Island and rode to Manhattan, covering the distance in sequence. Stops on the route were few and limited to government, medical or well-known landmarks selected to generate awareness. Schools were not on the radar since there was no compelling reason to focus on them.

That changed the day I stepped into Jerry's classroom and he planted the seed for student outreach. The school assembly programs I delivered developed a core of student activists committed to find a cure. These children altered the face of the Ride. With them, a new era dawned.

For the last several years, our largest single revenue stream has been from kids. They raised more for the Ride than any other source, including corporations. The school community has raised more than 1 million dollars to fight ALS. Hard to believe children out performed business. I suppose this reflects my emphasis on education and our extensive outreach program.

From our presentations last year, we selected five dozen schools to visit during the ten weekdays of the Ride. Patients arrive at these schools to a hero's welcome. Bands play, cheerleaders chant, signs wave and voices strain at the tumultuous receptions. The outpouring of love and compassion is overwhelming. The enthusiasm spreads among the students like dandelion seeds blowing in the wind. The experience has humbled and brought many PALS to tears. Gazing into the eyes of an innocent child as they tell our patients not to worry, they will find the cure, is powerful medicine.

The slow evolution of the Ride route to focus on schools began serendipitously. Pioneering schools hosting a Ride stop included my home district of Northport, my wife's district of Comsewogue and the district where I live, Miller Place. In addition, we went to North Babylon High School, where recently diagnosed PALS, Mary Murphy, was the librarian.

Flushed by the success of the 2004 Ride and buoyed by Jerry Shor's experience, I mailed letters to all of Long Island school principals requesting to make a presentation about the Ride and "Meeting the Challenges of Life." The first response was from Monica Caronia, principal of Nathaniel Woodhull Elementary School in the William Floyd District. In 2005, they became the template for the schools that followed.

Sadly, Mary died the next year and was only able to do one Ride. North Babylon High School, led by her dear friend

Barbara Brown, continued in her honor, raising $20,000 and set the gold standard for secondary buildings.

In subsequent years, more districts got involved. A nearby school of Northport, Burr Road Intermediate School, was the first blockbuster building without any direct link to ALS. Eileen MacAvoy hosted a presentation at her school, Cayuga Elementary. A colleague, Susan saw it. When she went home, she told her husband, the principal of Burr. Eileen invited the Hepplers to a Kick-Off celebration. Chuck Heppler heard about our work and the up-coming Ride. After meeting us, he invited me to give an assembly at his building. Following the presentation, they chose to make a difference. Even without a link to ALS, they raised $10,000 the first year, the highest total of any school building below high school. Burr continues to be among the highest raising schools every year.

Terri Maccia was an administrator at Burr Road. She left to be the building Principal at Marion Street School in Lynbrook. When she had the opportunity to be involved with the Ride, she jumped at it. Her building gave us a stunning reception.

"Chris and all the PALS with us today welcome. Our school conducted fundraising and we would like to donate $4,000 for your cause." Ms. Maccia said.

This past May, they went to more than $5,000, making them the highest elementary school on Long Island. Thank you Burr Road Intermediate for your far-ranging impact.

This story is incomplete without Mary Murphy's daughter, Jeanellen Murphy. Jeanellen broke her ankle and was unable to work which corresponded with the time her mother was struggling to finish the year as a teaching librarian. Jeanellen took advantage and spent her recuperation period helping her mom at school. Mary had the bulbar form of ALS, meaning it struck in the upper body region. She lost her ability to speak but remained able to walk and use her arms. Her daughter became her voice. After her mom died, Jeanellen began to rethink her life.

"Christine, I have decided to leave my job. I want to go back to school and become a teacher like my mom," she told my wife as they walked on the Ride.

The transformative experience assisting her mom and interacting with students taught the value of service. Five years after setting foot into her mother's classroom, Jeanellen entered her own. Completing her training quickly, she entered New York City's school system as a seventh grade English teacher in Washington Heights. It is an irony; Lou Gehrig lived in the Heights, not far from where she works every day.

Of course, she brought the Ride for Life! We have been unofficially adopted by her school. The last weekday of the Ride, we work with her school, Community Health Academy of the Heights (CHAH). Students enthusiastically escort us from Yankee Stadium in the Bronx over the Harlem River to their building in Upper Manhattan several miles away.

Their boisterous chants in English and Spanish made apartment windows rattle. They stir up their melting pot neighborhood with ALS awareness. The Heights is among the poorest communities in the city. Yet, they raise at least $10,000 every year!

Outside North Babylon, Mary's home school, CHAH's community of kids, staff and teachers is the highest fundraising building in the entire metro area. Those with the least give the most. A lesson for all....

Like the generations of student activists before them that I mentioned, these Long Island and city students are playing a part in finding a cure for ALS. When that day arrives, I hope these young people remember their role in making that possible. This book is a testimony to their effort.

Kids everywhere did everything to fight ALS. First graders wore pajamas to school so they can "put ALS to sleep." Students with parents queued up at beverage recycling machines getting nickels. Some piled up "pennies for patients." Buildings had halls bedecked with signed paper baseballs sold for a dollar. Brave principals and teachers held pie-throwing events. These young people and their school community have earned their spot in the story of "How ALS Was Cured."

I am proud to be a teacher. The students learned my life's lessons well.

The lesson I learned from this was throughout history, children have played important roles in making societal changes. They are a powerful source of action. For the ALS Ride for Life, young people are at the core of our organization and are responsible for a large portion of our donations.

Don't under estimate what they can accomplish.

God Is My Co Pilot

Because the ALS Ride is an awareness campaign traveling on the roads, it was imperative we had an eye-catching vehicle with informative banners to capture motorist's attention. On the first journey to Washington D.C., we enjoyed the use of a loaned recreational vehicle. Our daughter's boyfriend Glen Sheprow's family owned a motor home. His generous father allowed us to use it. Its sides made a perfect billboard. It displayed our mission in bold, large whitewashed letters. It was a simple but effective tool.

When we transitioned from D.C. to the New York area, we were fortunate to get a generous donation from a local business specializing in recreational vehicles, WES Trailers on Long Island. They lent us a motor home. We created a vinyl banner to display info about ALS and the Ride. The motor home became a rolling billboard and served as mobile command headquarters.

When the stock market crashed in 2008, the RV industry was hit hard. WES was unable to continue the loan. We were stuck and we scrambled for a replacement of the sign. Ray Manzoni secured a donation of a mobile sign truck. It was a fabulous vehicle with a sixteen-foot long by eight-foot high display area. We made a banner promoting the Ride. It became an annual feature. During another economic slowdown, the mobile sign trailer company fell on hard times. They too no longer donated a vehicle.

The search began for a permanent solution. Frank Timmons, a local friend, saw a trailer frame sitting behind a garage on a construction site where he was working. He inquired and found out it was from an old camping trailer.

"Chris, I have a great idea. I found a trailer. I think you should buy it," Frank said.

He wanted to purchase and build a platform to put up a sign. I agreed and bought it. A team of volunteers headed by Ed Weissbach built the sign platform. In a strange twist of fate, Ed's cousin Tommy was diagnosed and died from ALS several years later.

The trailer has become a fixture on each Ride. It is an iconic symbol of the event. Untold number of motorists and bystanders see the trailer pulled along the Ride route every year.

Generous supporters loan us their pick-up trucks to tow the sign trailer. The combined rig totals more than 40 feet long. A talented and dedicated squad of volunteer drivers pull the trailer wherever we go. Like pros, they negotiate congested streets and busy intersections as easily as a spider crosses its web.

On the 21st ALS Ride the trailer was on its way to rendezvous with everyone at the starting point at the Brooklyn Bridge for the last day. The trailer departed my house in Miller Place a half hour earlier because my handicapped van travels in the HOV lane of the LI Expressway and takes less time. A phone call interrupted our sleepy ride to the starting point.

Andy MacAvoy and his wife, Eileen, were ahead driving with the trailer. His wife made a frantic call to us and delivered shocking news. The conversation was difficult to hear with the signal often being lost. All we knew for certain was nobody was injured. The pickup truck my son-in law Rich loaned us was undamaged.

"The trailer broke away from the pick-up," she said. "It turned over and it was not useable."

Typical of most breaking news, its initial content was fragmented and confused. Eileen hung up because the police arrived. Dear God, I thought as we headed towards them.

Within a few minutes, we caught up. Both the truck and an upright trailer were on the right shoulder. My wife pulled off ahead. Andy walked over and filled us in.

"Something must have dislodged or sheared off the truck hitch," he said. "It let the trailer sleeve pull away from the truck."

We sat in the van listening in disbelief. "Then what happened?" my wife asked for the two of us. The hitch also had two safety chains. They were there for that possibility.

Andy said, "The trailer weight and speed snapped both chains."

The last protection was gone. Traveling in the middle lane and moving 50 miles an hour on the busy expressway, the trailer was now free. Andy could not believe what he saw next.

"I look off to the right and I see the trailer rolling by in the other lane!"

The wheel jack stand, used to crank the trailer coupling up and down off the hitch became the front axle for the speeding, out of control trailer. The small plastic wheel quickly broke, allowing the blunt bottom of the stand to scrap along the pavement.

"I'm surprised it did not dig into the pavement and make it flip over," I said.

We agreed, "Only a miracle prevented a disaster."

The trailer mysteriously pointed itself towards the shoulder. It missed the traffic in the right lane. The broken jack stand didn't dig deeply into the pavement. The trailer drifted safely to the shoulder and came to a stop.

"We gotta get it off," Andy said.

Now we faced the questions: How can we get it off the dangerous highway for repairs right away? Would it be ready for the last day of the Ride? The second unbelievable event occurring that day supplied the answer. An SUV pulled over in front of us.

As rain began, a man exited, pulled a hood over his head and walked past us to the trailer behind. I sat in my van unable to get out on the busy highway. I was burning up with curiosity wanting to know what the hell was going on. After an agonizing wait, my wife returned.

"The hooded stranger was an owner of a local trailer and hitch business!" she told me. "He saw us and stopped to help."

He understood exactly what happened and what we needed to get back on the road to bring the trailer home for repairs. In fact, he had the parts with him! Within minutes, the hitch was re-attached and the trailer moved safely off the highway for permanent repairs. We offered to pay for the part and something for his time.

"Nah, I don't want anything. I am glad I could help you guys." He went on saying, "Good luck with finding a cure."

He got back in his SUV and left. With nothing for me there, I also took off for the start point.

Tom Longo, a cracker-jack mechanic and all around tool guy, was about to leave his house for the start with his wife, Pat when he got a call. Andy explained the situation.

Tom replied, "No problem, I will stop and look at it. I'll bring stuff."

During Tom's drive in, the trailer was towed off the expressway to a safe spot where it could be thoroughly fixed. Tom arrived to work his magic. I got to the staging area and the call came.

"It is fixed and on its way in!" the voice on the other end announced. "It will be an hour late."

Andy resumed. He was not alone with Eileen. He had a third guest. God was his copilot.

The lesson I learned from this was not all angels have feathers and wings. They may assume many disguises. They come in all types of weather. They appear anywhere, like on the side of the road in the rain.

The First Amendment

To an educator, the voice is a powerful tool. It commands respect, informs and on occasion, inspires. The voice becomes our signature for the world. Losing it is catastrophic.

The diagnosis of ALS all but guaranteed that occurrence for me. I did not realize that at first. I was young, 44 years old, and I thought mostly about dying early and leaving all that I loved for eternity, whatever that meant. It was not until I recovered from the initial shock of the diagnosis that the grizzly details of how I would die began to come into focus. Chief among my many worries was losing my speech. It was the ultimate loss, isolating you from the world.

Of course, I knew and watched Steven Hawkins on TV. John Rather, a lawyer and fellow Long Islander, was the first PALS I met who lost his ability to talk. The experience of meeting John introduced me to my own perilous, winding journey to within.

We met when I was doing my ALS World Series baseball fundraiser. I went to visit so I could get to know him. I wanted to learn about his experience with the disease. His advanced progression startled me. A tube connected a vent to his trachea through a hole in his throat (tracheostomy). He lost the ability to talk as a result.

"Welcome," he said with his eyes. He grinned and winked.

"Hi John," I said. "Nice to get to meet you in person!"

John used an object called a letter board as a substitute voice. The alphabet was laid out on a sheet of paper in a grid of three rows numbered 1, 2 and 3. Two different background colors split the rows of letters down the middle dividing them into left and right. John used this board to compose words by selecting letters one at a time—sort of typing with your eyes.

To pick a letter, John blinked. For yes, usually twice in order to differentiate it from an ordinary blink. No blink automatically meant no. To use the board, the caregiver held it in front of John.

"Green?" the caregiver asked (or whatever the first color was) meaning that the first letter was in that colored section.

If not, the caregiver knew it must be in the other colored area. They continued searching to narrow down possible letter choices even more.

"Row one?" John was asked, to determine which row his letter resides in. When the row was correct, John blinked for yes. Now, with only 6 letter choices left, the caregiver read each letter in the row.

"Yes," John blinked on hearing the correct letter.

Letter by painful letter, word by tedious word, the caregiver methodically worked to unlock his message.

"It is nice to meet you also," he blinked out.

"Wow," I expelled, twinged with guilt that I spoke so effortlessly. "John, that is incredible."

Inwardly, I grimaced and cringed at the thought that would be me someday. I think John tried to smile with a sense of pride for his small victory.

He brushed off my compliment saying, "It's easy."

As he did, I envisioned him in court passionately fighting for his client. Now he fought just to communicate.

"Damn disease," I muttered under my breath.

The next time I went to visit, instead of the letter board, he used an impressive piece of equipment only emerging into the market. John was a pioneering user of a different kind of augmentative speech device, one that employed the latest innovative technology. Because he was educated and affluent, he was able to keep abreast of the newest equipment becoming available for use with ALS.

"Hey John," I said as I came in his room to find him sitting behind a computer screen on his chair.

"Good to see you," his synthesized voice answered. His focus shifted back to his device. I stood over him and watched.

His device originated with the military. The modern Air Force now had planes that flew at unimaginable speeds. Fighter jet pilots screamed across the sky covering a mile every 2 seconds. There was no time to look away from the windshield and gaze down at the instrument panel to see critical gauges. Each second counted when a missile was rocketing towards them or locked in a dogfight with an enemy. Engineers had to keep up with speed. They needed to develop a way to see critical information about the plane without the pilot looking down. Over time, they designed a 'Head's Up Display' enabling pilots to see critical data displayed right on their helmet's visor. This revolutionary technology changed the world.

The disabled community eventually benefited from the "Heads Up Display" development. The technology became the basis of eye-controlled computers. John used an early version of one. It attached to his chair and was set to a precise distance and angle from his eyes.

"It has two tiny infrared cameras that trained a beam at my pupils," he explained.

"Impressive," I admitted.

He went on, "The beam reflects back and the receivers next to them registered where my eyes looked. Through a series of calibrations, all spots over my whole monitor get calculated."

As John gazed across his screen cameras followed his gaze point. Through the application of mathematical formulas, the software in the computer was able to predict wherever he looked.

Through the genius of programming, designers turned this raw data into a useful tool. They created an integrated language package combining virtual keyboards with selection techniques to accommodate a range of disabilities (blink, dwell time or switch inputs). Voice synthesizers produced the final spoken word. John was able to 'type and speak' with his eyes.

John said, "It is pretty amazing. I am getting fast."

"You work that like you were born with it." I complimented him.

He brushed it off, "It is not hard to do." He went on, "I can't use it outside or in bright lighting. That is a big limitation."

We spent the better part of an hour "talking" about the eye-controlled computer. I wanted to know everything. By the time I left, I was grateful to know the option existed.

I thought a lot and worried about losing my voice. Since arm movement was the first to go, handwriting was not an option. Still, I would rather talk than use my arms, although either were precious choices to lose.

Steady and slow over 20 years, I listened to my voice deteriorate.

"Say that again, Chris, I didn't catch that," people told me.

My family and friends innocently tried to reassure me about my declining speech. Their lack of honesty frustrated me. I could handle the truth; it was the uncertainty that upset me. I wanted to plan for my future and learn to cope with loses. I wanted honest feedback, not well-meaning denial. Maybe they were projecting their own difficulties accepting my future.

Because of my voice, I began using a volunteer to deliver the bulk of my school presentations in about 2012. I retained some key power lines to deliver myself. ALS's relentless progression continued and the quality of my words forced me to use the eye-controlled computer in 2014. By 2017, I reluctantly stopped using the phone except with family or some friends. They saw me often enough to know my voice. I grew more reserved in social settings. This was a difficult transformation for me.

Outside of school, I struggled trying to talk to the public. It was clear that my days of speaking, beyond an intimate few words here or there, was sadly over. I suppose being able to adjust over years eased the heartache of losing my voice—as intimate a companion as my shadow. Oddly, within my head my voice remains as vibrant and clear as ever. It is only when

I verbalize my thoughts that undecipherable, alien words emerge from my mouth.

I grieved in my downtime, which was not too often. I had plenty of time to accept it. I lasted 20 years after seeing my first in-person assistive speech device before I advanced to a point where I had to use an eye control computer and voice synthesizer. I wrote much of this book with my device. I think an ancient Mesopotamian scribe chiseling a cuneiform message on a clay tablet could write my book faster. It's done after 12 months of staring for hours, blurry eyed at my 15-inch monitor.

I admonish myself not to complain, since most PALS reach this sad milestone in a fraction of the time. Nonetheless, it was-and still is- a bitter pill to swallow. Even now, I refuse to surrender totally, forcing those around me to decipher the garbled junk I try to pass off as words. Nancy Vermillion and Pat McGuinness typed the early part of this book. The latter came to my house for over 13 years to listen to me dictate. Pat worked as a secretary in Comsewogue School District and knew about me through my wife, Christine, who often interacted with her. Nancy attends St. Louis DeMontfort Church with me. She replied to a help needed blurb in the church bulletin and helped me for years as well.

The patient pair listened, resorting to an occasional guess. What fueled them I wondered? Did they put themselves in my situation? Sometimes I just smile to ease the stress on their part.

"It is like playing charades," I sometimes joked, "Maybe I could invent a party game and rent myself out to play charades with the guests using me as the clue giver?"

I think it would be a great fundraiser, I cannot figure out why no one agreed. The smile and jokes are great safety valves. They release the tension and lets us find humor in everything. My friends want so badly not to disappoint or frustrate me.

"You are so patient," many people tell me. They do not know the me they don't see. I am far from a saint.

When I cannot breathe, am in pain or must go to the bathroom, the patience evaporates. I must be honest. I do shout even if garbled, "Come on get this done already!" I am not nice if they do not understand right away. Like a parent hearing an angry infant, the words may not be understandable but the message is loud and clear. I am pissed.

Without my voice, I still move on. Like John decades ago, I cannot use my device outside. I must resort to the faithful and simple letter board. It is fail proof. Some things never change.

At least I can still exercise my right to speak, albeit slowly, with the help of this system. That makes me a fortunate man. There are ALS patients laying in hospital beds who are unable to write or speak. They are trapped and frightened, unable to make their needs known.

Why does this happen? Hearing impaired and non-English speaking receive interpreters. The Constitution provides certain inalienable rights, including the right to speak. Further, federal laws over the last two decades address discrimination based on disability.

"I demand we be treated as equals," I say to everyone.

A desperately ill ALS patient (along with a host of similar illnesses such as strokes) who are unable to express their wishes have the same rights as everyone else. Perhaps the Constitution applies only up to the hospital door.

This violation of basic human rights requires immediate resolution. At a minimum, eligible patients need direct access to a skilled letter board interpreter. As with a DNR, NPO or any other advisory chart, they must display a letter board in the patient's room. Hospitals must provide one. In my opinion, the first amendment says so.

Speech is freedom. Communication is the connection to the outside world. We all have a right to speak and be heard.

"I want to be able to speak, even if it is only one blink at a time."

The lesson I learned from this was that communication is a fundamental essential component of living. People go to great lengths to maintain it. Never be afraid to speak up. Your opinions matter.

Acknowledgements

We are grateful to many people who played an important role in making our book possible

- Lorraine Rau who saw the need I had and became my first volunteer in my home office working until she moved south to warmer weather
- Pat McGuiness is our longest volunteer helping every Tuesday since 2005
- Nancy Vermillion, a volunteer from our parish who replied to a plea for help in the church bulletin and helped for ten years

Our terrific caregivers who do everything in their power to help me 'live' and be productive despite ALS

- Amanda Moriarity has been here at my side for almost six years
- Tiana Quintero a bit over five years
- Lena Tizio for over one and a half years
- Marquita George for over one year

Those who were instrumental in my evolution as a writer

- Brian Heinz a colleague, naturalist, author and friend of 40 years

- Irene Nadler my first authentic audience who listened patiently
- Anne Edmonds my writing group leader
- Al Jordan who gave me confidence as a writer
- Liza Frenett a reporter who advised and critiqued my work

About the Author

Chris Pendergast

We are childhood sweethearts. In the sixties I was a paper-boy in a luncheonette, neither of which are common today. The store sold and when I met the new owner along with his family, my teenage eyes bulged out of my head. It was love at first sight. I was 16 and she was 13. We married eight years later in 1973.

At Fredonia State University College, I received my BA in secondary education. Then my teaching career began in 1970 in the Northport school district. I earned an MA from Stony Brook University in 1976. For the last half of my career I became a facilitator for the Gifted and Talented Program. Shortly after creating the Habitat House nature science center 1991, I was stricken with ALS.

Following the diagnosis, my wife and I chartered a new course through uncharted territory. We became ALS warriors. I continued working until 2003. Simultaneously initiated an aggressive advocacy campaign. The ALS Ride for Life originated in 1997. The School of Medicine at Stony Brook University awarded me an honorary Doctorate of Science in 2005 for my work on ALS. I have been advocating and working ever since.

Christine Pendergast

I often simply introduce myself as the wife of Dr. Christopher Pendergast. However, I earned my BS in Education at Brockport State University College in 1973 and an MA from Stony Brook University in 1992. For 32 years I was a Physical Education teacher . Over those years, I taught every grade level. In addition to teaching, I was a coach for a variety of sports. I ended my career as Dean of Students for the high school.

In addition to teaching, I was a union activist volunteering for several different positions. I served as President of our local Teachers Union. I loved my career and union work.

Chris's diagnosis pushed us in a different direction. I also assumed the role of advocate as well as an ALS caregiver. My role as a caregiver was not new. As the eldest of five siblings, I had responsibilities caring for someone from early on. For my work on behalf of patients and their caregiver spouses, I received a Woman of Distinction Award issued by the New York State Senate in 2007. The longevity of my experience with Chris enabled me to develop a unique, valuable perspective. I organized a caregiver's support group in 2011 to address their unmet, specialized needs. It established an environment for safely expressing feelings without judgement. In 2019, the ALS Association of Greater New York selected me as a recipient of the first Eleanor Gehrig Caregiver Award.

With support, I enjoy my hobbies of golf, city trips with my friends and an annual solo vacation to Aruba. I enjoy reading and gardening. He encourages me to live my life to the fullest. Alongside my husband, I helped raise our two children Melissa and Buddy. We were blessed with our grandson

Patrick in May 2007. He is the best grandson anyone could ask for.

My proudest accomplishment is a loving marriage of 46 years. For 27 years, it was an 'open' marriage where I was forced to share my husband with another partner, one that I despised. ALS has taken the body of the man I fell in love with, but not his personality, romanticism, determination or strength.

God is good all the time. All the time, God is good.

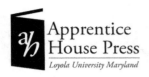
Apprentice
House Press
Loyola University Maryland

Apprentice House is the country's only campus-based, student-staffed book publishing company. Directed by professors and industry professionals, it is a nonprofit activity of the Communication Department at Loyola University Maryland.

Using state-of-the-art technology and an experiential learning model of education, Apprentice House publishes books in untraditional ways. This dual responsibility as publishers and educators creates an unprecedented collaborative environment among faculty and students, while teaching tomorrow's editors, designers, and marketers.

Outside of class, progress on book projects is carried forth by the AH Book Publishing Club, a co-curricular campus organization supported by Loyola University Maryland's Office of Student Activities.

Eclectic and provocative, Apprentice House titles intend to entertain as well as spark dialogue on a variety of topics. Financial contributions to sustain the press's work are welcomed. Contributions are tax deductible to the fullest extent allowed by the IRS.

To learn more about Apprentice House books or to obtain submission guidelines, please visit www.apprenticehouse.com.

Apprentice House
Communication Department
Loyola University Maryland
4501 N. Charles Street
Baltimore, MD 21210
Ph: 410-617-5265 • Fax: 410-617-2198
info@apprenticehouse.com•www.apprenticehouse.com

CPSIA information can be obtained
at www.ICGtesting.com
Printed in the USA
JSHW051322150920
7932JS00003B/132

9 781627 202572